Atlas of Practical Cardiac Applications of MRI

Atlas of Practical Cardiac Applications of MRI

Atlas of Practical Cardiac Applications of MRI

Guillem Pons-Lladó, MD. Director, Cardiac Imaging Unit, Cardiology Department, Hospital de la Santa Creu i Sant Pau, Universitat Autónoma de Barcelona, Barcelona, Spain.

Francesc Carreras, MD. Cardiac Imaging Unit, Cardiology Department, Hospital de la Santa Creu i Sant Pau, Universitat Autónoma de Barcelona, Barcelona, Spain.

Xavier Borrás, MD. Cardiac Imaging Unit, Cardiology Department, Hospital de la Santa Creu i Sant Pau, Associate Professor of Medicine, Universitat Autónoma de Barcelona, Barcelona, Spain.

Maite Subirana, MD. Director, Unit of Congenital Heart Diseases, Cardiology Department, Hospital de la Sant Creu i Sant Pau, Universitat Autónoma de Barcelona, Barcelona, Spain.

and

Luís J. Jiménez-Borreguero, MD. Cardiology Department, Hospital Principe de Asturias, Alcalá de Henares, Madrid, Spain.

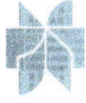

SPRINGER-SCIENCE+BUSINESS MEDIA, B.V.

Library of Congress Cataloging-in-Publication data is available.

ISBN 978-94-010-5931-2   ISBN 978-94-011-4544-2 (eBook)
DOI 10.1007/978-94-011-4544-2

Printed on acid-free paper

Contents

Medicine has been characterized during the second half of the twentieth century by a succession of spectacular advances in all fields. With respect to diagnostic methods, imaging techniques are required by clinicians with increasing frequency. Cardiology is one of the disciplines which has been most intensely affected by this phenomenon, on which different interesting phases may be distinguished. First, during the decade of the sixties, the clinical tasks were supported only by plain radiography and the electrocardiogram. The introduction of angiohemodynamic techniques in the following decade represented the first stage in the modernization of diagnostic cardiology, which was not accompanied by a similar development in the field of non-invasive methods, such as phonocardiography and pulse recordings, that continued to be used as an auxiliary tool. The introduction of Doppler echocardiography and isotopic methods in the eighties represented a radical change in this sense, providing the clinical cardiologist with real noninvasive methods to document the diagnosis in practically all aspects of cardiac disease, except for the anatomy of the coronary arteries. The widening of the horizons of angiohemodynamic techniques toward interventionalism has, at the same time, caused the global map of the applications of diagnostic methods to shift toward the point of equilibrium that we are familiar with today, one that makes cardiology one of the most highly technological disciplines.

With this overview, we have seen, in the nineties, the arrival of magnetic resonance imaging (MRI), the introduction of which has represented for other specialties the same revolution that cardiology underwent with the introduction of ultrasound. Proof of the utility of the cardiac applications of MRI is to be found in the profusion of published reports and articles by dedicated groups of investigators on the subject, as well as in the efforts these groups are making in translating their experience with MRI to the clinical grounds, which have presently allowed the technique to attain an interesting place in practical cardiology. There is no doubt about its present utility or the immediate future that awaits it, although there are aspects which influence its practical application and that should be known when evaluating its role among cardiac diagnostic methods.

MRI makes its appearance in a historic moment in which the field of cardiology is already served by a suitable amount of imaging techniques, and MRI will inevitably be compared to them in terms of competition. On one hand, MRI is relatively expensive and unavailable, since it is shared by different disciplines. On the other hand, it has in its favor the characteristics of an imaging technique of excellent resolution, reproducibility and wide field of vision without interference from paracardiac structures. But the aspect that probably makes it the most attractive is the perspective that it holds for the near future: by taking advantage of all its modalities, it can be considered as a technique offering in an integral manner all the diagnostic information that is required for the majority of cardiac patients, data which, at present, it is necessary to obtain by the combination of various diagnostic methods. It is in fact recognized that today MRI can be considered as a method of reference for the estimation of the dimensions of cardiac chambers, the measurement of ventricular mass, ventricular function and the study of blood flow. Now that research into its capacity to study miocardial perfusion and the very anatomy of coronary arteries is yielding promising results, it is not an overstatement to affirm that this future is now approaching. Under these conditions, the above mentioned limitations, all of which are of a strategic nature, will not represent an insurmountable obstacle.

This perspective has brought about the presentation of this book, based on the experience initiated by our group of Cardiac Imaging of the Department of Cardiology of the Hospital de Santa Creu i Sant Pau. An idea we had in mind when we approached this task was the peculiar situation that presently characterizes cardiac MRI: on one side, there is a large body of information in specialized journals produced by groups with a high degree of expertise and working with the most advanced technology; on the other hand, however, the degree of implementation of cardiac MRI in practice may be considered as definitely low, even in centers where suitable conventional MRI units are available. It is our personal feeling that this paradoxical underdevelopment of a technique with such a high potential value derives from

the fact that the practising cardiologist sees MRI as a complex method rendering information that is in some way redundant or, at best, that the technique is at present just an innovative research tool. This is, in our view, a false perspective, that will ultimately prevent or delay the access of the cardiologist to an important source of clinical information, even when only the most basic equipment is available. It is time, thus, to initiate this approach in practice.

To help in this respect we have attempted in the present book to provide technical information about MRI, the bases of its cardiac applications, accepted indications in daily practice, with examples of its capabilities, and a vision of its possibilities at present under research. A glossary of terms and a reference bibliography concerning each subject have been included with the objective of improving its didactic nature. We hope that this book will contribute to increase the knowledge of cardiac applications of MRI among those cardiologists and also radiologists interested in the field.

It must not be forgotten that adequate practice with cardiac MRI is always the result of close collaboration between cardiologists and radiologists. Therefore, the authors of this course, all of us cardiologists, wish to recognize their radiologist colleagues, whose continued orientation and willingness to help have been crucial in order to acquire the experience that is reflected in this work. We also wish to mention the centers where the authors have obtained the imaging studies which illustrate this work, as well as the members of the radiological teams that, in each case, have collaborated with us:

Servicio de Radiodiagnóstico, Hospital de Santa Creu i Sant Pau de Barcelona (Drs J. Llauger and J. Palmer).

Centro de Resonancia Corachán, Clínica Corachán de Barcelona (Drs. J.M. Caussa, C. Alexander and J. Álvarez-Moro).

Centro de Resonancia Magnética Balear, Clínica Femenía de Palma de Mallorca (Drs. D. Taboada and A. Lanuza).

Centro SERDIASA, Clínica San Camilo de Madrid (Drs. J.M. Alfonso and M. Padrón).

Axial plane: horizontal transverse plane.

Breath-hold: voluntary interruption of respiration necessary for the correct acquisition of some ultrarapid sequences.

Cine MR: series of gradient-echo images obtained in consecutive phases of the cardiac cycle and displayed in a continuous loop sequence.

Coil: element of the MRI system that generates the radiofrequency pulses used to excite the study subject (transmitting antenna), or that also receives the echoed pulses returned by tissues (receiving antenna). The same coil can act as both transmitter and receiver, or there can be two independent coils, one for each function.

Coronal plane: vertical frontal plane.

Echo planar imaging (EPI): technique enabling the acquisition of an image by means of a single radiofrequency excitation in a time on the order of milliseconds.

Fast low-angle shot: gradient-echo sequence that uses short repetition times and reduced matrix, thus allowing the acquisition of images in less than a second.

Field strength: degree of intensity of the magnetic field generated by the system magnet (measured in Tesla units).

Field of view (FOV): dimension of the study window.

Flip angle: value reached by the precession angle when stimulated by a specific radiofrequency pulse.

Free induction decay (FID): name given to the radiofrequency signal emitted by the protons of tissue during relaxation after having been submitted to radiofrequency excitation at resonance frequency in the presence of an intense, external magnetic field.

Frequency encoding: a process which enables the location of a point along one of the axes of the study plane: along with phase encoding, it defines the position of this point in the study plane.

Gadolinium (chelated): paramagnetic contrast agent of intravascular and extracellular distribution that produces a change in T1 and T2 relaxation times of the tissues, thus improving their contrast in the images.

Gating: coupling between slice acquisition of a sequence and any cyclical physiological signal: ECG; respiration, peripheral pulse.

Gradient echo (GE): MRI technique by which adequately contrasted images are obtained of dynamic structures and of blood flow. Due to the short repetition times employed, it is possible to include various excitations in one cardiac cycle time, which enables the acquisition of dynamic cine MRI sequences.

Imaging time: duration of a complete study.

Interslice gap: distance, which does not appear in the image, that separates contiguous slices of a sequence.

Magnet bore: element contained in the core of the MRI system that generates the intense magnetic field on which the technique is based.

Matrix: number of information units (voxels) that constitute the image.

Multi-phase: any sequence in which each slice is obtained in multiple phases of the cardiac cycle.

Multi-slice: any sequence in which multiple contiguous slices are obtained simultaneously.

Oblique plane: plane with a certain degree of angulation over any one of the standard planes (axial, coronal or sagittal).

Phase encoding: a process which enables the location of a point along one of the axes of the study plane: along with frequency encoding, it defines the position of this point in the study plane.

Pixel size: dimensions (in mm) of the information unit in the two-dimensional representation of the image on the screen. Image resolution depends on pixel size, which varies according to field of vision and matrix.

Precession angle: angle between the vector axis of the external magnetic field and the rotation axis of the hydrogen proton.

Pulse sequence: series of consecutive excitations and receptions, its analysis resulting in the acquisition of images with any one of the MRI techniques.

Radiofrequency: fragment of the electromagnetic spectrum that includes waves with frequencies under 10^{12}. The radiofrequency waves used in MRI have frequencies of 10 to 100 MHz.

Radiofrequency pulse: brief radiofrequency signal emitted to excite the protons of the hydrogen atoms of the study subject.

Relaxation time: time required for the return to a resting state of the hydrogen protons after a radiofrequency pulse excitation. Longitudinal relaxation or T1 is the time it takes them to return to the basal precession angle. Transverse relaxation time or T2 is the time elapsed until the energy acquired by phase coherence, in which protons are under the influence of an external radiofrequency pulse, is lost.

Repetition time (TR): interval between the emission of two radiofrequency pulses.

Sagittal plane: vertical antero-posterior plane.

Scout image: initial plane of rapid acquisition used to locate the first sequence.

Segmented-k-space: fast imaging technique based on the acquisition of grouped lines of information (segments) instead of the line-by-line method used in conventional techniques, this reducing the acquisition time of an image to a matter of seconds.

Signal void: area of absent signal due to the flow characteristics in a specific region of the slice plane: it appears in instances of high flow rate or of turbulence in gradient-echo sequences.

Signal averaging or number of excitations (NEX): number of repeat measurements required for a sequence to be obtained with adequate definition of the images.

Signal-to-noise ratio (SNR): relation between the signal intensity from tissue structures and the background image noise, upon which image quality depends.

Single phase: any sequence in which one or various slices are obtained, each one in a different phase of the cardiac cycle.

Single slice: any sequence in which the images are obtained from a single slice.

Slice thickness: width of the slice.

Slice: section of the study subject under study.

Spatial resolution: ability to discriminate between two different structures in the image, depending on the field of view and the matrix size.

Spatial presaturation: excitation of previous adjacent slices to the one under study with the aim of avoiding unwanted flow signals.

Spectroscopy: technique that permits the acquisition, in an area of a specific tissue displayed in the MR image, of the spectrum of concentrations of an element (usually phosphorus) according to the different chemical compounds in which it is present.

Spin echo (SE): MRI sequence that provides images of adequate contrast between tissues and blood flow, as no signal is elicited by rapidly moving structures.

Tagging: MRI technique in which equidistant crossing lines are magnetically preselected in the ventricular myocardium, allowing dynamic myocardial wall changes to be tracked during the cardiac cycle.

Tesla: standard unit of magnetic field strength.

Time of echo (TE): time interval between the radiofrequency pulse emission excitation and the reception of the radiofrequency signal emitted by the tissues.

Ultrafast sequences: techniques applying information acquisition strategies designed to reduce the total time spent in the process of imaging.

Velocity mapping: process which permits the analysis of flow velocities present in the study plane.

Voxel: tridimensional unit of the MRI matrix that integrates the two dimensions constituting the pixel with the thickness of the slice.

Wash-out effect: effect by which the blood flowing in a direction perpendicular to the slice plane produces a characteristic absence of signal (signal void), in the spin-echo technique, due to the fact that the excited blood leaves the slice plane well before the echo signal is read.

Basics of cardiac magnetic resonance and normal views

1

X. BORRÁS-PÉREZ

F. CARRERAS-COSTA

G. PONS-LLADÓ

1.1 Definition and Physical Basics

a. Definition and historical background

Magnetic resonance (MR) is a physical phenomenon which is produced in the nucleus of some atoms basically consisting of the emission of a radiofrequency (RF) signal generated by the nucleus itself after having been stimulated by RF pulses in the presence of a strong external magnetic field. The computerized analysis of the emitted RF signal may be used both for the study of the chemical composition of tissues, a technique known as MR spectroscopy, and to obtain anatomical images, this constituting the clinical magnetic resonance imaging (MRI) methods.

The physical phenomenon of nuclear MR was discovered in 1946[1]. The first clinical images obtained by this technique were published in 1973[2]. The explosion of computer technology in the eighties allowed the development of the first commercial equipment, the earlier reports on cardiac applications being published in 1983[3]. Today, the technique of cardiac MRI is continuously expanding[4,5], as is demostrated by the amount of clinical reports on its application, which were over 400 during 1998, some of them coming from expert committees summarizing the present indications of the technique[6] or addressing the particular requirements for an optimal application of MRI in cardiology[7].

b. Physical basics

Elemental particles such as protons and electrons, which constitute matter, exhibit an electric charge and undergo a continual spinning movement. They therefore generate a magnetic field. Of these magnetic fields, the stronger one is that originated by the protons of the atomic nuclei. Those elements with an atomic nucleus possessing an even number of protons show a null net magnetic charge, as the individual charges tend to mutually neutralize one another. On the other hand, elements with an odd number of protons show a definite magnetic charge, their nucleus acting as a small dipolar magnet, the basic condition required for the phenomenon of MR. Hydrogen is an atom with a single proton that is widely present in all structures from the body in the form of water (H_2O), which is the most used element in human MR, especially in imaging techniques.

• Formation of the magnetic vector of the body

The magnetic fields of the hydrogen atoms of the body are oriented at random, the global magnetic field of the body being thus zero (Figure 1.1). In order to elicit the MR phenomenon we must first arrange the magnetic fields of the hydrogen atoms, which is accomplished by placing the body under the influence of an intense continuous magnetic field (field strength of 0.5 to 2 Tesla). The application of such a strong magnetic field results in the alignment of the dipolar magnets of the hydrogen atoms with the longitudinal axis of the field and in either a parallel or antiparallel orientation. Since the parallel alignment results in a better entropic condition than the antiparallel position, a somewhat larger number of nuclei arrange themselves in the former alignment. This small difference between the nuclei in parallel antiparallel positions causes the weak resultant magnetic vector that is originated in the body when submitted to an intense external magnetic field (Figure 1.2).

Actually, the magnetic dipoles do not align in a strictly static position (parallel or anti-parallel) under the external magnetic field, but they exhibit an oscillation, much like spinning tops, describing a movement called precession, which causes them to deviate slightly from the axis of the external field on a specific angle called the angle of precession. The precession frequency of these nuclei depends on the external magnetic field, and is unique for each level of field strength, being called the Larmor's resonance frequency. The resonance frequencies for the hydrogen atom under the effects of field strengths varying from 0.5 to 2 Tesla oscillate between 20 and 100 MHz. These values fall within the range of the RF waves of the electromagnetic spectrum. Fortunately, the human body can be submitted to them without any risk of ionizing effects.

• Emission of radiofrequency in resonance

When a hydrogen nucleus under the influence of an external magnetic field receives an energetic charge by means of a RF wave pulse emitted at its resonance frequency, a deviation of the angle of precession is produced (Figure 1.3). This deviation is proportional to the duration and intensity of the pulse of the RF wave. An RF signal that produces a deviation of the precession angle of 90° with respect to the axis of the external magnetic field (conventionally known as the z-axis) is called a 90° pulse. When the RF signal is interrupted (Figure 1.4A), the nucleus returns to the basal state, with the previous precession angle, and the excess energy generated in this process is liberated in the form of a new RF wave at the resonance frequency (Figure 1.4). The liberated RF wave is known as FID (Free Induction Decay). The detection of this RF wave by means of an appropriate antenna (induction coil) constitutes the base for both the technique of MR imaging as well as for MR spectroscopy.

The return of the hydrogen nucleus to the basal state following the cessation of the RF pulse is called relaxation. The intensity of the RF wave signal emitted during relaxation has vectorial characteristics and can be considered as constituted by a longitudinal component, aligned with the axis of the external magnetic field (z-axis), and by a transverse component (xy-plane). Changes in the longitudinal vector can be attributed to the displacement of the spin axis of the nucleus toward the axis of the external field, accompanied by a decrease in the precession angle and the resulting increase in the vector of longitudinal magnetization. The time required for the longitudinal vector to return to its value prior to stimulation by the RF pulse is called longitudinal relaxation time, or T1, and can be plotted on a graph of signal intensity with respect to time (Figure 1.5A). This return occurs exponentially in tenths of a second, and while it is a function of the intensity of the external field, it also depends on the proton composition of the medium. Thus, longitudinal relaxation time is clearly different for tissues with different percentages of water.

The transverse vector, which is the representation of the xy-plane (perpendicular to the axis of the external magnetic field) and its value reflects the energy secondary to the coherence in the spin phase of the different hydrogen atoms. In the absence of RF

FIGURE 1.1

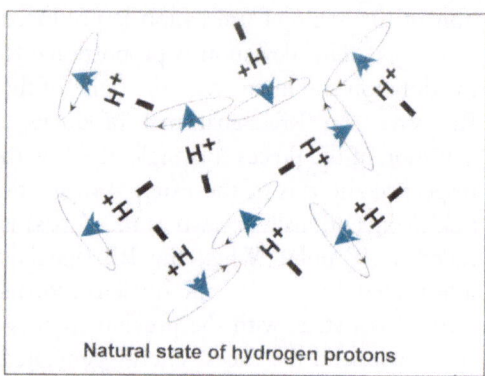

Natural state of hydrogen protons

FIGURE 1.2

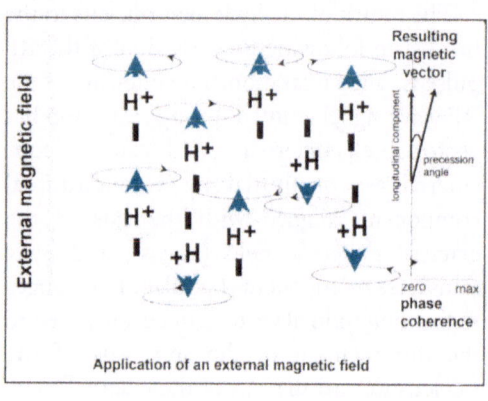

Application of an external magnetic field

FIGURE 1.3

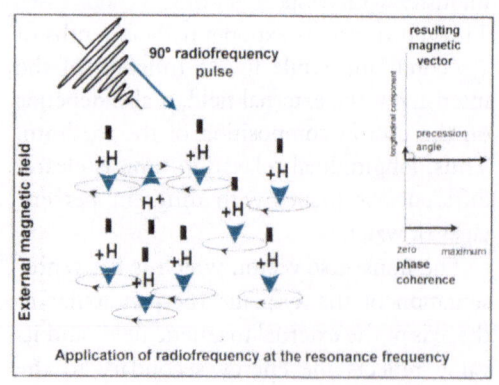

Application of radiofrequency at the resonance frequency

FIGURE 1.4

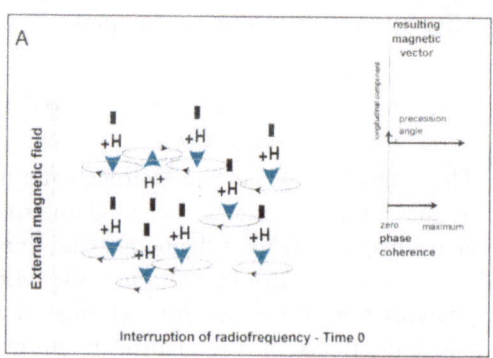

Interruption of radiofrequency - Time 0

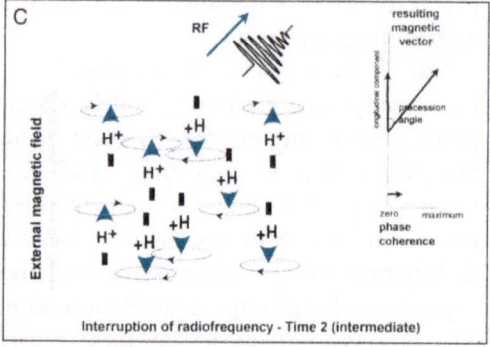

Interruption of radiofrequency - Time 2 (intermediate)

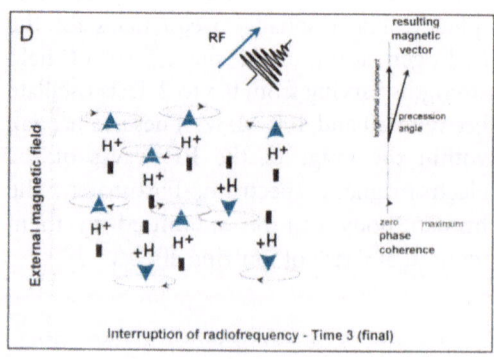

Interruption of radiofrequency - Time 3 (final)

stimulation, each hydrogen nucleus spins with a different phase. The resultant value is then zero, but when an RF pulse is applied, the nuclei couple in a phase (all spinning together at the same time) and the transverse vector is then maximum. When the RF signal is interrupted this coherence and, as a result, the energy contained in it, are lost. The loss of energy due to phase coherence is known as transverse relaxation, and the time that elapses until a position of equilibrium is regained is called transverse relaxation time or T2. The decrease in energy in the transverse plane is an exponentially decreasing function that reaches zero in hundredths of a second (Figure 1.5B). Transverse relaxation is conditioned by two factors: first, due to the existence of physical inhomogeneities in the external magnetic field and, second, by tissue composition. In order to obtain an image allowing an appropriate tissue characterization, the influence of inhomogeneities in the external magnetic field over transverse relaxation must be neutralized. To accomplish this aim, a second RF signal pulse with a phase shift of 180° is applied. Since it is supposed that the inhomogeneities of the magnetic field are fixed, adding a signal of 180° is equivalent to multiplying by a factor of –1, which eliminates the nonvariable components while retaining only the influence of the tissue composition in the signal. Transverse relaxation time is very sensitive to the presence and type of other atoms that surround hydrogen originating the resonance signal. Thus, it varies greatly according to the different tissues, but it is practically unaffected by the intensity of the external magnetic field.

In summary, after applying a 90° RF pulse, a second refocalizing pulse of 180° is applied and, finally, the RF signal emitted by the tissues (echo signal) is detected (Figure 1.6). The interval between the 90° RF pulse and the echo signal is designated as time of echo (TE). The 180° RF refocalizing pulse is applied halfway through the interval of the 90° pulse and the emission of the RF echo signal. The information is read during the emission of the echo pulse from tissue.

• Formation of resonance images

Values of the longitudinal and transverse vectors can be measured by means of induction coils acting as antennas. Maps can be drawn from these numerical values and, when coded in a scale of greys, an MR image is formed. Many cycles of excitation and relaxation are necessary in order to detect these values. The interval between two of these cycles (two RF pulses) is called time of repetition (TR). The comparison between the signal intensity of different tissues, which we call contrast, can be increased by varying the TR and the time between the RF pulse emission and signal reception (TE).

Signal intensity is influenced by values of T1, T2, and density of the hydrogen protons in the tissue. Images based on T1 relaxation time (T1 weighted) must be obtained by means of short TR and TE (Figure 1.7). When imaging the heart this causes surrounding fat to appear with a bright white color, the pulmonary air and the blood which flows

---

F. 1.1.   Random distribution of the magnetic dipoles of the hydrogen atoms under natural conditions.

F. 1.2.   Hydrogen atoms under the influence of a strong external magnetic field. The magnetic dipoles are aligned with the external magnetic field, most of them in the same direction (parallel) and some in the opposite one (antiparallel). The difference between both directions causes the resulting magnetic vector diverging from the direction of the vector of the external magnetic field with the precession angle. The hydrogen atoms spin in different phase, the value of phase coherence being thus null.

F. 1.3.   Application of a RF pulse at resonance frequency of sufficient energy to increase the precession angle to 90° (90° pulse). Most of the magnetic dipoles orient themselves in an antiparallel direction. It can also be observed how the increase in the precession angle reduces the value of the longitudinal component of the resulting vector. The coherence phase value reaches its maximum as the majority of the atoms spin at the same time.

F. 1.4.   (A) Cessation of the RF pulse: the longitudinal component of the resulting magnetic vector is minimum and the value of the phase coherence is maximum. (B) The hydrogen atoms change from antiparallel to parallel position with the emission of energy in the form of a RF pulse at resonance frequency: the precession angle is reduced, increasing the longitudinal vector, and phase coherence starts to decrease. (C) Intermediate time in the process of relaxation: a progressive increase in the longitudinal vector value and a decrease in the transverse vector of phase coherence may be observed. (D) End of relaxation and of RF emission: the atoms return to the parallel position (in the same proportion as prior to stimulation), the original precession angle is recovered, and the maximal value of the longitudinal component of the resulting vector and the disappearance of phase coherence are attained.

rapidly to appear as a dark color ("black blood") and the cardiac muscle showing an intermediate intensity. In order to display the differences between tissues in T2 weighted images, much longer TR and TE than those for T1 weighted images must be used, due to the fact that it is a decreasing exponential function with longer relaxation times (Figure 1.8). This may constitute a limitation in the analysis of cardiac structures due to their rapid constant movement, which means that images obtained with long TR and TE are affected by artifacts.

• Locating the slice plane

Submitting the body to a uniform magnetic field causes all the protons to spin at the same frequency. To obtain information about a specific plane, it is necessary to add a second magnetic field whose intensity varies along one of the body's axes (e.g. the longitudinal axis), which creates a magnetic gradient. In this way, the resonance frequency of the nuclei varies along the body axis (in our example, the protons of the head will have a different resonance frequency from those of the neck, and these, in turn, from those of the thorax, and so on). Thus, protons from each level can only be excited by RF waves coincident with the particular resonance frequency. Therefore, in order to locate a particular plane of study, we must apply an RF wave of the same frequency as that of the area of interest we wish to explore. The remaining areas will be unresponsive to this excitation. In this way, we will be able to obtain slices orthogonal to the established magnetic gradient (in our example, planes transverse to the longitudinal axis of the body). Additionally, if slices at a superior or inferior level are required, it is then necessary to adjust the RF wave to the resonance frequency of the desired area. The narrower the band of frequencies of the RF wave, the narrower the thickness of the transverse slice will be. Obviously, changing the orientation of the gradient allows slices with different orientations to be obtained, thus covering all the potential space planes without moving the patient.

• Location within the slice plane

In order to locate each one of the points within the selected slice plane, a phase gradient and a frequency gradient in the reading are applied, both of them oriented orthogonally to the magnetic gradient that defines the slice plane. For example, considering a defined longitudinal magnetic gradient along the body allowing a transverse slice plane to be obtained, the phase gradient could be used to give the location in an antero-posterior direction, while the frequency gradient in the reading would give the location in a left-to-right direction. Each one of the data matrix points which form the image is defined by a single phase and frequency combination that permits its spatial location. During the formation of the spin echo, the receiving antenna coil, connected to an analog-digital converter, collects information on frequency, phase and amplitude for each point delimited by the triple gradient, all the points contributing to the recomposition of the data matrix being obtained consecutively (Figure 1.9).

Data acquisition time varies according to repetition time (TR), the size of the image's matrix (which determines the phase-encoding steps) and the number of excitations programmed for phase encoding. Time is in the order of minutes to obtain an image sequence. Any movement during this time, whether voluntary from the subject, or due to rhythmic changes of heart position or of the lungs, will provoke phase and frequency alterations which will be registered as artifacts. In order to minimize them, it is important to synchronize the ECG as well as respiration during image acquisition, which will significantly prolong the examination time.

1.2 Technical Modalities

There are diverse modalities of the MRI technique useful in the field of cardiology, each one of them providing particular modes of information with definite applications in the study of the cardiovascular system (Table 1.1).

Essential in any case is that the machine be equipped with a system for synchronizing (gating) the signal emission with the patient's ECG: since the formation of an MRI image results from a series of consecutive acquisitions, an accurate timing of these excitations with respect to the cardiac cycle is mandatory

FIGURE 1.5

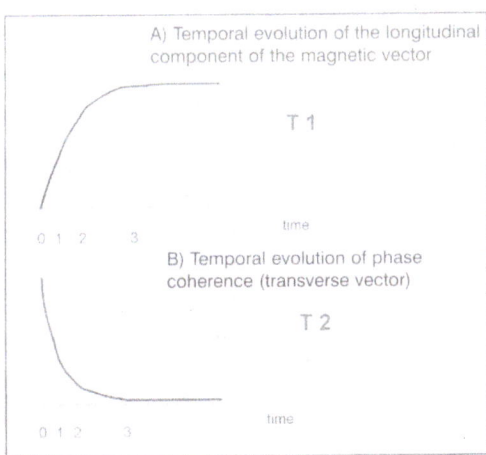

FIGURE 1.8

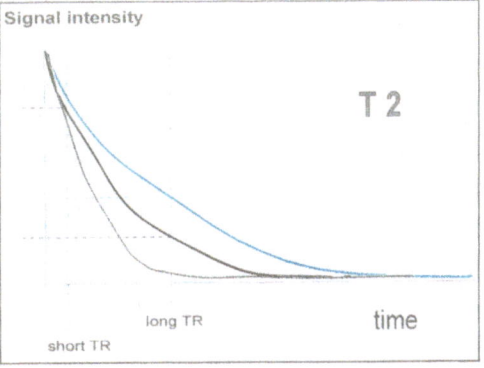

FIGURE 1.9

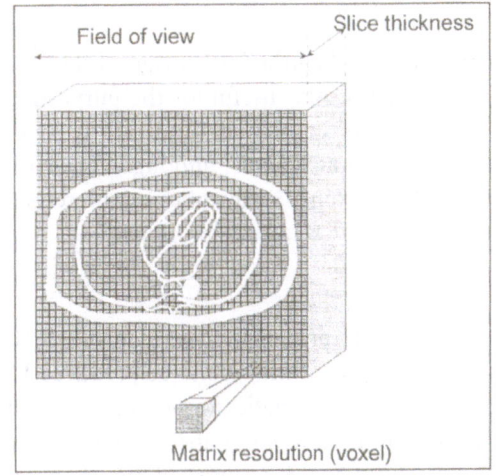

FIGURE 1.6

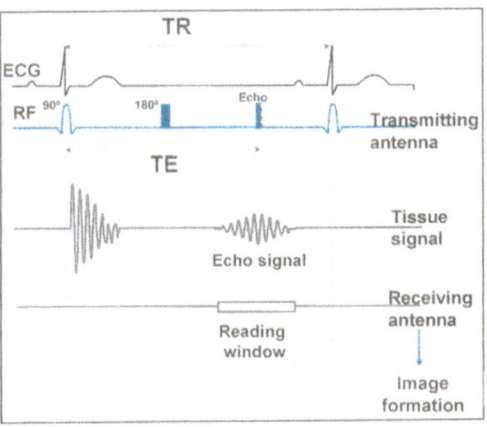

FIGURE 1.7

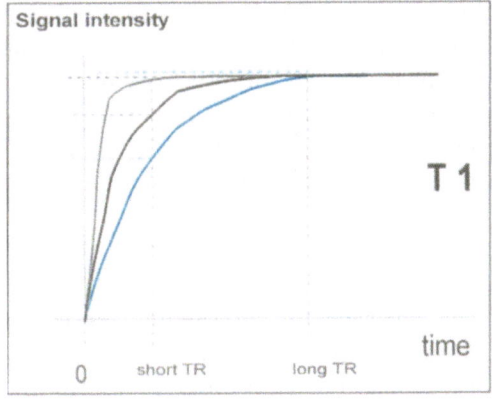

F. 1.5. Temporal evolution of the longitudinal component of the resulting magnetic vector (A) and temporal evolution of the vector which represents phase coherence in the spin of hydrogen atoms (B): 0 to 3 correspond to the time phases referred to in figure 1.4.

F. 1.6. Excitation sequence in the formation of a spin-echo image. Gated with the R wave of the ECG, a 90° RF pulse is emitted which generates a tissue response signal (not read). At the TE/2 time, a refocalizing pulse of 180° is emitted. At a TE interval after the 90° RF pulse a tissue signal (echo) is produced, which is read by the receiving antenna for processing and image formation. ECG: electrocardiogram. RF: radiofrequency. TE: echo time. TR: repetition time.

F. 1.7. Repetition time (TR) and tissue differentiation in T1 weighted images: short TR discriminate intensity values of the T1 signal from different tissues; long TR allow tissues to recover their maximum initial value of signal intensity and no differences between them are detected.

F. 1.8. Repetition time (TR) and tissue differentiation in T2 weighted images: short TR do not discriminate intensity values of the T2 signal from different tissues; the diverging curves of tissue signal intensities along time allow its adequate detection when using long TR intervals.

F. 1.9. Elements defining the image in MRI.

Table 1.1 Technical modalities of MRI and their applications in cardiovascular studies

Technique	Information	Application
Spin-echo	Static tomography	Morphology
Gradient-echo	Static/Dynamic tomography	Morphology/Function
Fast gradient-echo	Static/Dynamic tomography	Morphology/Function Angiography/Perfusion
Velocity mapping	Flow curves	Flow/valvular studies
Myocardial tagging	Myocardial mechanics	Myocardial function
Spectroscopy	Chemical tissue composition	Metabolic studies
Echo-planar	Static/Dynamic tomography	"Real time" studies

in order to obtain a final image of an adequate quality. Also useful for the purpose of image quality is synchronization with respiratory movements, although this considerably prolongs study time and, therefore, this procedure is not used routinely.

a. Spin echo

Available in practically any general MRI system, the spin echo technique produces T1 or T2 weighted static images of excellent resolution used to study the morphology of cardiovascular structures. This type of sequence provides a signal intensity of the structures which depends on their histological constitution, the signal reaching maximum intensity in those rich in adipose tissue with a high concentration of hydrogen ions[8]. Circulating blood, on the other hand, presents a characteristic absence of signal, due to the wash-out phenomenon (time elapsed between the two excitations by acquisition in which the spin echo modality is based, which allows the blood volume excited during the first excitation to leave the study plane during the second one)[9]. This results in a marked natural contrast between the vessel walls or the endocardium and normal blood flow ("black blood" technique) (Figure 1.10) although, even under conditions of normal blood velocity, it is not infrequent that erratic signals of intraluminal flow may appear in some slices, due to the fact that blood volume from previous slices may have been saturated. This phenomenon occurs naturally in cases of stasis or abnormally slow circulation.

The acquisition of a T1 weighted spin echo sequence requires 5 to 6 minutes and results in a series of between 6 and 12 contiguous slices, depending on TR, which is, in turn, dependent on the spontaneous heart rate of the patient.

b. Gradient echo

This technique of acquisition provides images of adequate definition for morphological studies and also offers the possibility of dynamic studies when a series of between 12 and 30 static images of the same slice acquired in different phases of the cardiac cycle are displayed in a continuous loop format (cine MRI)[10]. This is possible due to the short TR values the technique allows, on the order of 50 ms, although the acquisition strategy entails five minutes for each sequence. The technique is also extremely sensitive to blood flow. Only one excitation is employed in this modality, the blood flow appearing with a high signal intensity ("bright blood" technique) (Figure 1.11). Although gradient echo sequences produce a lower contrast of static structures than that of spin echo, they do have an additional advantage, such as the visualization of blood turbulence, which gives rise to a characteristic phenomenon known as "signal void" which contrasts naturally with the blood circulation of laminar flow[11].

c. Fast gradient echo

The relatively time-consuming process of obtaining images by means of the previously mentioned modalities has prompted the development of rapid sequences[12]. Based on strategies of reducing TR and TE parameters, a category of techniques known as fast gradient echo (turbo-FLASH, GRASS, SPGR) allow an image to be obtained in less than 1 second and can be implemented on conventional systems. Also, an innovative modality in which the whole array of spatial frequencies that correspond to an image (k space) is acquired in the form of portions (segments) permit the acquisition of a series of images in 12 to 16 seconds. This can be accomplished during a period of voluntary apnea of the patient (breath-holding), by which interferences due to respiratory movements are significantly reduced (Figure 1.12)[13]. Although the use of these rapid sequences inevitably implies a trade-off between time of examination and spatial resolution, their practical application is rapidly spreading due to the fact that time saving is crucial in certain studies, as is the case when transient events are to be captured (i.e. contrast perfusion studies), when the presence of some arrhythmias complicates the application of conventional sequences, or in the troublesome time-consuming process of imaging the coronary arteries.

d. Specialized techniques

There are modalities that require a specific software program that, although available for most of the systems, is not included as a basic option. This is the case of myocardial tagging programs[14], velocity mapping[15] and MRI angiography[16]. Since they are not routinely used in all general radiology departments, we will refer to them only occasionally.

e. Techniques under clinical investigation

Finally, other modalities require important modifications, hardware included, such as spectroscopy[17] and the technique of echo planar[18]. The latter is of great interest, since it permits the acquisition of all information of k space in a single heart beat, providing images with acquisition times on the order of milliseconds ("real time"). Although they are not in use at the present in most centers, their potential is under active clinical research.

1.3   Study Methodology: Normal Anatomy

a. Technical equipment
- A high field strength giant solenoid superconducting magnet in the range of 0.5 to 2.0 Tesla.
- RF magnetic field gradient coils used to determine the position, thickness and orientation of the imaged slice.
- Central computer to control the analysis of the MRI signal and the formation of images.
- Console control to operate the MRI system: programming of the study, signal emission and image control.
- Software programs for the different applications.
- Printing system for radiographic films.

b. Medical personnel
- Radiology technician in charge of the machine.
- Radiologist or cardiologist, ideally both working together as a team, in charge of study strategy design and image evaluation.

c. Preparation of the patient

MRI is a prolonged examination (20 to 60 minutes) that requires total patient co-operation. Claustrophobia, which occurs in a small percentage of cases, can lead to the suspension of the study. Patients should be informed that they will have to remain motionless during the examination and that the machine generates loud noise. Young children or nervous patients should be sedated or given anaesthesia by an anaesthesiologist. The patient should avoid excessive swallowing, and respiration should be as regular as possible, avoiding large diaphragm movements (sighs, cough, etc.).

• Improving image quality

Respiratory movements affect largely image quality (Figure 1.13), and although they can be partially avoided with a respiratory gated system, this method prolongs the examination to such a point that it is not used in practice. New synchronizing devices have

14

FIGURE 1.10

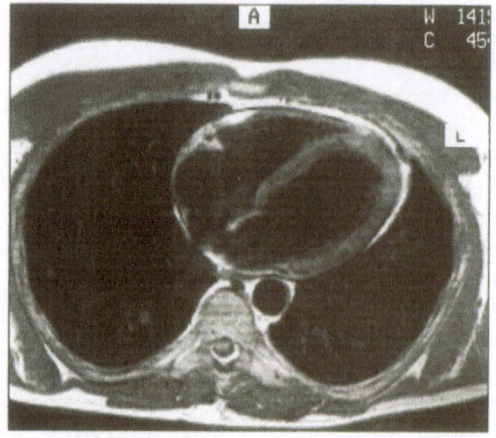

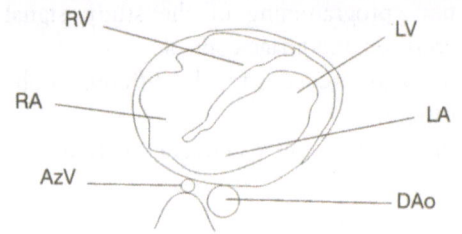

FIGURE 1.12

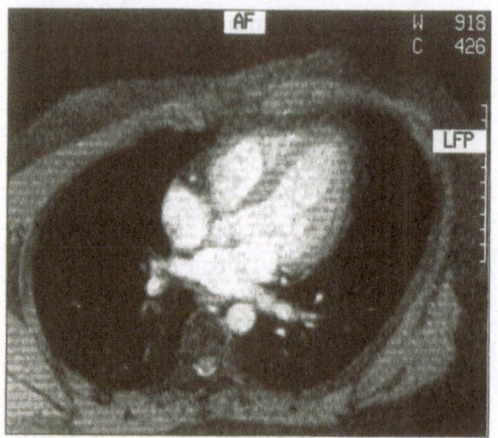

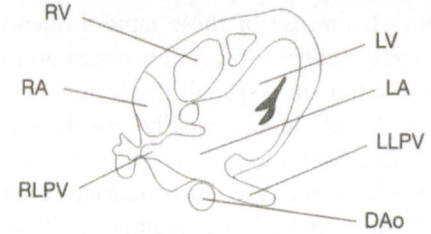

FIGURE 1.11

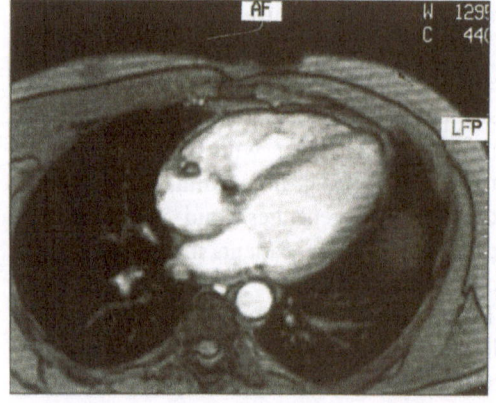

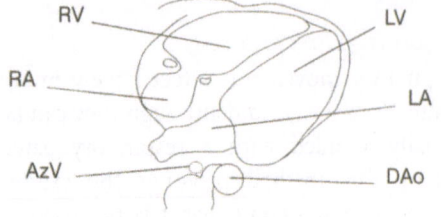

FIGURE 1.13

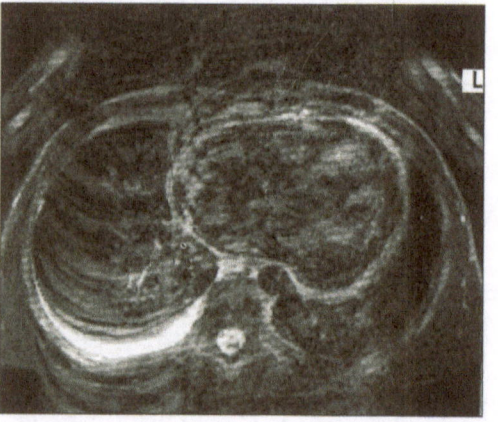

been developed, gating image acquisition to respiratory movement by means of a re-positioning of the signals that form the image in coordination with movements of the diaphragm, determined by a system of navigator-echoes processed by the machine. Although the most comfortable position for the patient is prone, supine position would be preferable, since it reduces the generation of artifacts secondary to respiratory move-ment. The use of breath-hold sequences, if the patient cooperates in order to successfully accomplish them, avoids those artifacts due to respiratory movement at the same time as it significantly shortens examination time.

The presence of frequent premature beats or atrial fibrillation with irregular heart rhythm is also an inconvenience to obtain good quality images. Normal respiratory sinus arrhythmia can even be problematic, espe-cially if the patient breaths slowly and deeply.

• *Artifacts*

Ferromagnetic material and paramagnetic substances generate important image artifacts due to local changes in the magnetic field around them, which are most pronounced in the images obtained by gradient-echo sequences. In operated cardiac patients suture wire of the sternum or valvular prostheses are a frequent cause of artifacts that are otherwise circumscribed around the object that generates it and, thus, the evaluation of the rest of the image is not hampered.

• *Safety considerations*

MRI is an examination technique that does not produce lesions in biological tissue. The existence of a mild thermal effect has been documented, but it does not affect even sensitive tissues such as testicular or corneal. The contraindications of the study arise from the effect of the magnetic field on magnetic or metallic prosthesis or implants (Table 1.2). Thus, in the case of patients with cardiac diseases it is important to be aware that those with implanted pacemakers or defibrillators should not undergo the examination, since the powerful magnetic field can interfere with the electronic components and cause them to function abnormally, leading to the possibility of producing serious arrhythmias. Likewise, in patients with thermodilution catheters the electromagnetic field can cause overheating due to induction currents gener-ated by the metal content of the catheters, which can cause serious burns, especially at the cutaneous insertion area of the catheter.

Nevertheless, in the specific case of patients with a cardiac disease, neither the metal clips used to identify aorto-coronary by-pass grafts, suture wire in the sternum nor vascular-coronary endoprosthesis (stents) represent a contraindication for an MRI study. It is also not contraindicated to study patients with valvular mechanical prosthesis, except in the case of the old Starr-Edwards model (Pre-6000), which has a high ferro-magnetic content. The small torsion force that may be produced in the prosthesis, due to the effect of the magnetic field, is much less than that which is generated by the mechanical force of the heartbeat. Concerning other new kinds of materials, the tendency of those to be implanted in the body is to avoid ferromagnetic material, precisely in order to prevent risks during MRI examinations. However, it is advisable to consult up-to-date revisions of the listings of prostheses and implants published periodically in specialized journals in case an MRI examination might be contraindicated[19].

F. 1.10.   MRI in spin echo technique showing the characteristic signal absence of normal blood in the interior of the heart chambers and the aorta, as well as the high signal intensity generated by paracardiac adipose tissue; the ventricular myocardium has an intermediate signal intensity. AzV: azygous vein; DAo: descending aorta; LA: left atrium; LV left ventricle; RA: right atrium; RV right ventricle.

F. 1.11.   Image using the gradient echo technique, with opposite characteristics to those of spin echo, in which the higher signal intensity corresponds to blood flow. AzV: azygous vein; DAo: descending aorta; LA: left atrium; LV left ventri-cle; RA: right atrium; RV right ventricle.

F. 1.12.   Image obtained by a fast gradient echo technique (segemented-k-space) during breath-hold. DAo: descending aorta; LA: left atrium; LLPV: left lower pulmonary vein; LV: left ventricle; RA: right atrium; RLPV: right lower pulmonary vein; RV: right ventricle.

F. 1.13.   Example of a poor quality spin echo image caused by signal artifacts due to respiratory movements and poor electrocardiographic synchronization.

Table 1.2 Contraindications for the practice of a magnetic resonance study

Pacemaker, implanted defibrillator or neurostimulator
Intracranial iron clips
Metallic intraocular foreign body
Metallic fragment near a vital structure (projectile)
Cochlear implant or hearing aid
Starr-Edwards mitral valve prosthesis, model 6000 or earlier
Claustrophobia
Critical patient with a Swan-Ganz catheter
Pregnancy (relative: teratogenic effect not demonstrated)

• Physiological gating for image synchronization

In order to obtain conclusive images of the cardiovascular system by means of MRI, it is necessary to synchronize (gate) image acquisition to the cardiac cycle. This requires that the electronic controls of the machine receive some type of physiological signal. The signals used for synchronization are the ECG or the pulse wave signal.

The most appropriate gating signal is the ECG R wave, since it permits one to either program or to determine accurately the relation between MR images and the cardiac cycle. It is common knowledge that the surface ECG signal is obtained by means of electrodes placed on the skin which detect the electric activity of the heart, which generates a variable magnetic flow. When the patient is placed inside the machine, where there is a very powerful magnetic field, respiratory movements and abrupt changes of magnetic gradient that occur during the examination cause the generation of potentials induced between the electrodes. They are superimposed on the base ECG tracing, creating artifacts which can cause the signal to be unrecognizable. In addition, another artifact, especially if the machine is 1.5 Tesla or higher, may be added, a phenomenon known as the magneto-hydrodynamic effect. When the blood cell particles with an electric charge (ions) move in a direction perpendicular to the magnetic field, they create additional electric potentials in the cardiovascular area. This gives rise to the formation of a prolonged electric pulse which usually superimposes itself on the ECG T wave. Occasionally the intensity of the artifact is such that it creates a signal of the same amplitude as the R wave, causing problems in the mechanism that detects the synchronization signal.

Artifacts generated in the ECG signal can become a significant practical problem, sometimes difficult to solve, but they can be minimized by taking into consideration some rules:

- Electrodes should be placed on those areas of the body that are the most likely to remain motionless, taking special care to avoid respiratory movements.
- Excessive distance between electrodes should be avoided.
- Care should be taken so that the potentials induced among the electrodes are parallel to the magnetic flow lines of the machine in order to minimize its amplitude.
- Stretch out the electrode wires to the maximum.

In order to avoid the risk of the electrodes absorbing energy and heating up, which could damage the skin, electrodes that have been specially designed for use in MRI machines should be used. In order to avoid damage to the eyes, which are especially sensitive to excessive radiofrequency irradiation, electrodes and their wires should not be placed near the head.

If acquisition of a proper register of the ECG signal becomes problematic, the pulse wave signal amplitude can be used as a synchronizing tool. Nevertheless, it should be kept in mind that the temporary definition of the pulse wave is not as precise as the ECG R wave. To detect the pulse wave amplitude, capillary optic sensors are generally employed, and they should be placed on the fingertips, as long as they are well perfused.

With this technique artifacts are basically produced by the movements of the extremities. The recording of a signal of low amplitude is usually due either to thick skin, which impedes the correct function of the optical mechanism, or to poor blood circulation. Above all it is necessary to use appropriate sensors with electric wires that do not act as antennae in order to avoid overheating and the risk of cutaneous lesions. Excessive compression of the digital sensor must be avoided, since prolonged examinations might cause fingertip ischemic lesions.

d. Normal MRI anatomy

In spite of the different commercial models of MRI systems, each one with its specific software, there are common pulse sequences for cardiovascular imaging, as well as anatomical image study planes that one should become familiar with. Although MRI allows slice planes to be obtained in any direction of the space, it is advisable to perform the study in a standard way, which facilitates appropriate image analysis.

Once an initial localizing scout image, generally on a coronal orientation, has been obtained, it is advisable to initiate the examination with a standard, multislice T1 sequence in the axial thoracic plane that includes, as much as possible, the longitudinal axis of the thorax. This will display the anatomical relation of the cardiovascular structures to the rest of the thoracic ones in the standard axial plane. These planes will be used as a base for the planning of the following study planes. It is not recommended to start by programming on the scout plane rapid single-slice sequences in order to locate a specific plane as various attempts are normally necessary, and more time is consumed than that used in a conventional multislice spin echo sequence. Also, excessive reliance on oblique planes or double obliquities can create serious difficulties with the interpretation of the relations of anatomical structures. The more complicated the anatomical structure to be studied is (e.g., a complex congenital heart disease), the more necessary it is to undertake the study methodically, including standard orthogonal planes (transverse, sagittal and coronal) that are easily interpreted, in order to avoid confusion upon analyzing anatomical relations.

• Transverse or axial plane (Figures 1.14–1.21)

It is especially useful to study the anatomical relations of cardiovascular structures by analyzing images at consecutive levels.

• Sagittal plane (Figures 1.22–1.27)

The sagittal plane allows the analysis of the right infundibulum and the main pulmonary artery in longitudinal views. It also permits a suitable study of the atrial septum, both cava veins and the thoracic descending aorta.

• Coronal plane (Figures 1.28–1.32)

It allows the analysis of the relation of the trachea and the main bronchi to the cardiovascular structures. The left ventricular outflow tract and the vascular structures can be adequately seen.

In order to selectively study the cardiovascular anatomical structures, especially cardiac chambers or the great vessels along their anatomical axes, planes with one or two obliquities are necessary.

• Sagittal oblique planes

A view displaying the whole thoracic aorta is obtained by a plane programmed on an axial slice encompassing the planes of the ascending and descending portions of the aorta (Figures 1.33 and 1.34).

A two-chamber view of the left ventricle (vertical longitudinal) is obtained when a plane including the base and the apex of the ventricle is planned on an axial view (Figures 1.35 and 1.36).

• Four-chamber plane: double angulated plane (Figure 1.37)

This horizontal longitudinal view of the heart is obtained from the previous one, programming a new plane that includes again the base and the apex of the left ventricle

• Left ventricular short axis: double angulated plane (Figure 1.38)

It is defined from an image plane orthogonal to the longitudinal axis of the left ventricle, starting either from a sagittal oblique plane or from a four-chamber plane.

References

1. Purcell EM, Torrey HC, Pound RV. Resonance absorption by nuclear magnetic moments in a solid. Physical Rev 1946; 69: 37.

2. Lauterbur PC. Image formation by induced local interactions: examples employing nuclear magnetic resonance. Nature 1973; 242: 190–1.

FIGURE 1.14

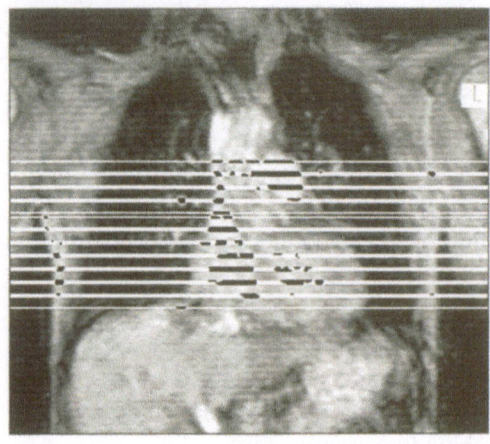

FIGURE 1.16

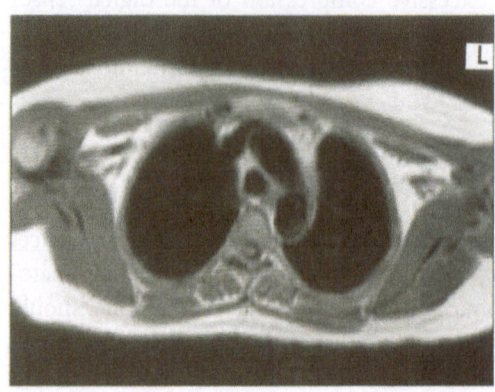

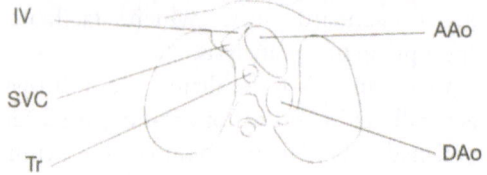

FIGURE 1.15

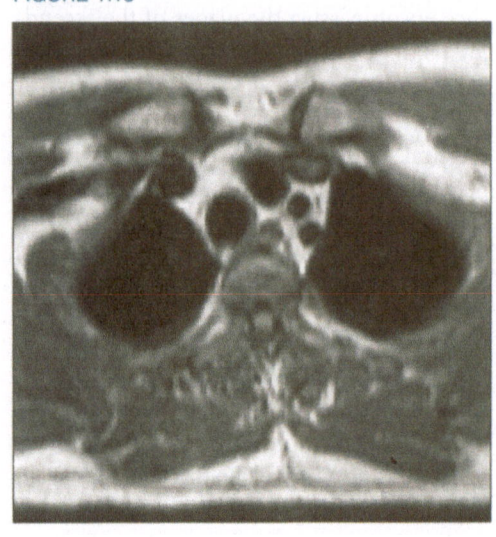

FIGURE 1.17

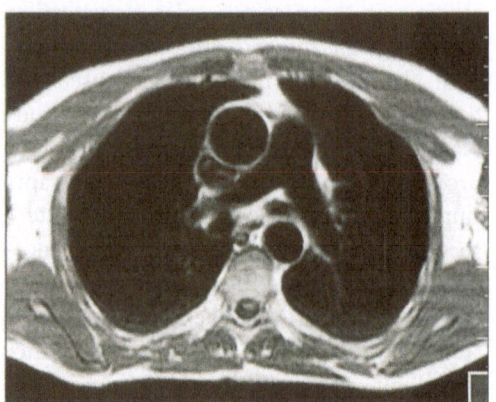

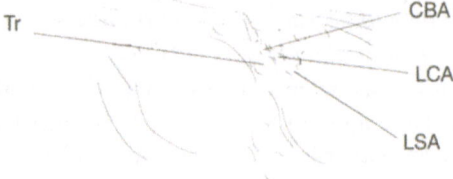

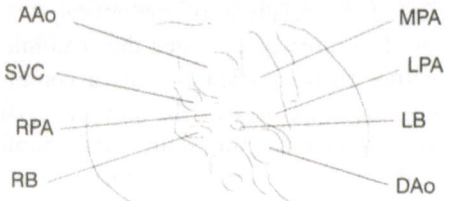

F. 1.14. Programming of an axial spin echo sequence on a coronal localizing plane used as anatomical reference.

F. 1.15. Axial plane at the level of supra-aortic arterial vessels. CBA: common brachiocephalic artery; LCA: left carotid artery; LSA: left subclavian artery; Tr: trachea.

F. 1.16. Axial plane at the level of the aortic arch. AAo: ascending aorta; DAo: descending aorta; IV: innominate vein; SVC: superior vena cava; Tr: trachea.

F. 1.17. Axial plane at the level of great vessels. AAo: ascending aorta; DAo: descending aorta; LB: left bronchus; LPA: left pulmonary artery; MPA: main pulmonary artery; RB: right bronchus; RPA: right pulmonary artery; SVC: superior vena cava.

FIGURE 1.18

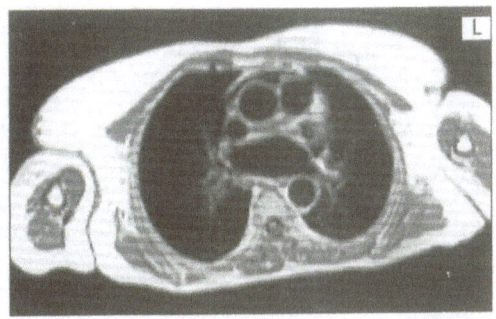

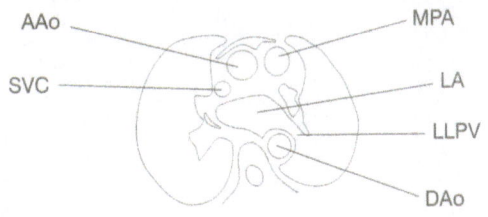

FIGURE 1.20

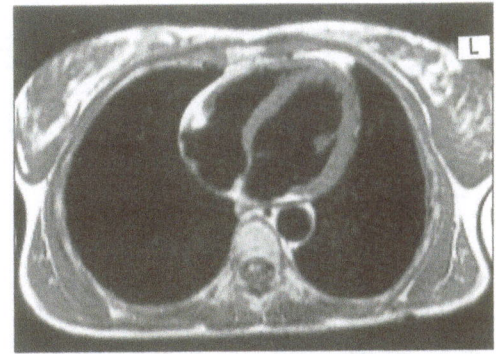

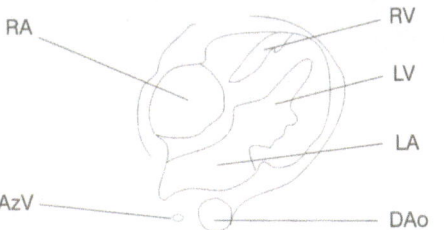

FIGURE 1.19

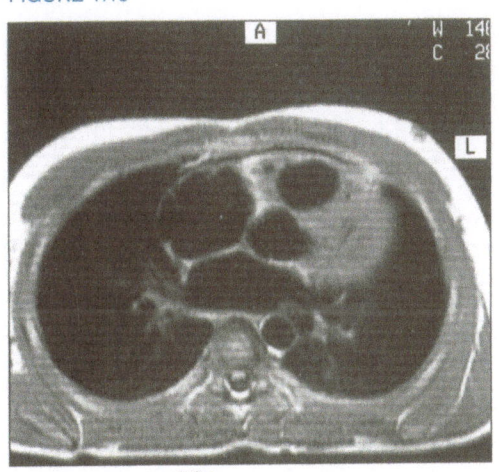

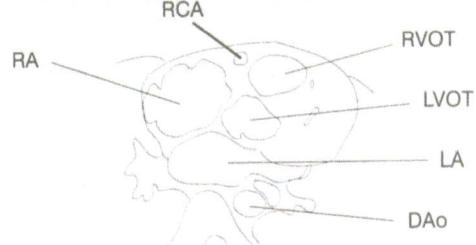

FIGURE 1.21

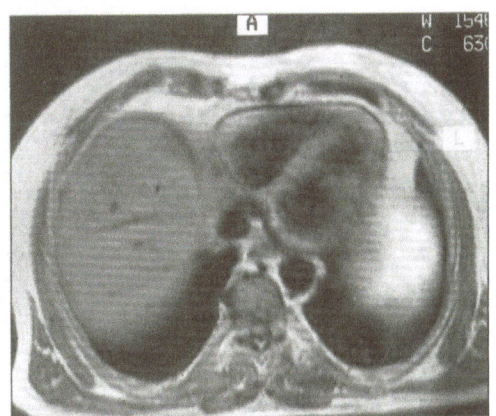

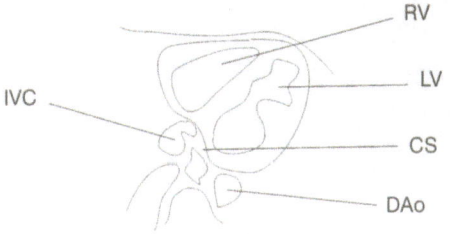

F. 1.18. Axial plane at the level of left atrium. AAo: ascending aorta; DAo: descending aorta; LA: left atrium; LLPV: left lower pulmonary vein; MPA: main pulmonary artery; SVC: superior vena cava.

F. 1.19. Axial plane at the level of ventricular outflow chambers. DAo: descending aorta; LA: left atrium; LVOT: left ventricular outflow tract; RA: right atrium; RCA: right coronary artery; RVOT: right ventricular outflow tract.

F. 1.20. Axial plane at the ventricular level. AV: azygous vein; DAo: descending aorta; LA: left atrium; LV: left ventricle; RA: right atrium; RV: right ventricle.

F. 1.21. Axial plane at the level of the inferior vena cava. DAo: descending aorta; CS: coronary sinus; IVC: inferior vena cava; LV: left ventricle; RV: right ventricle.

FIGURE 1.22

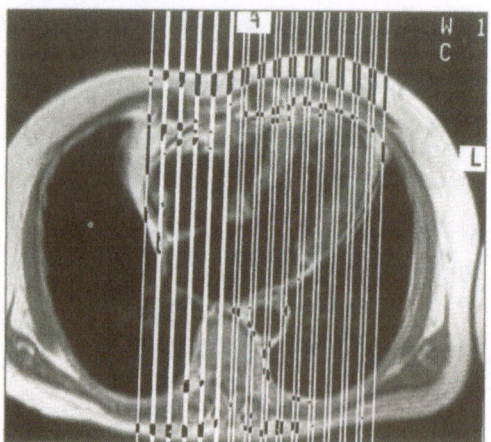

FIGURE 1.24

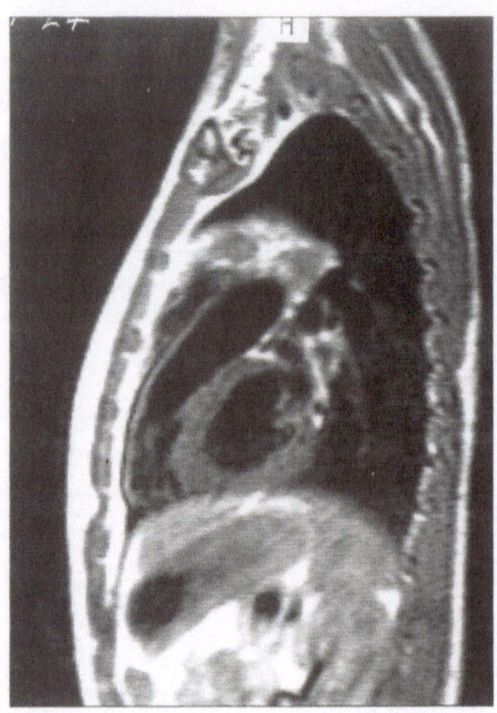

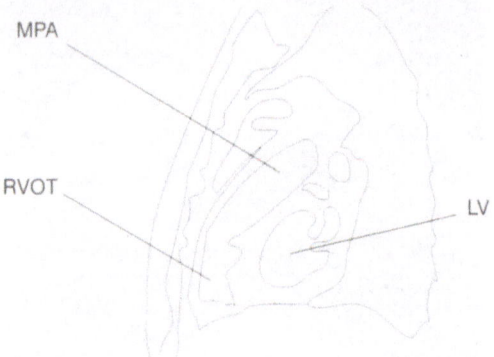

FIGURE 1.23

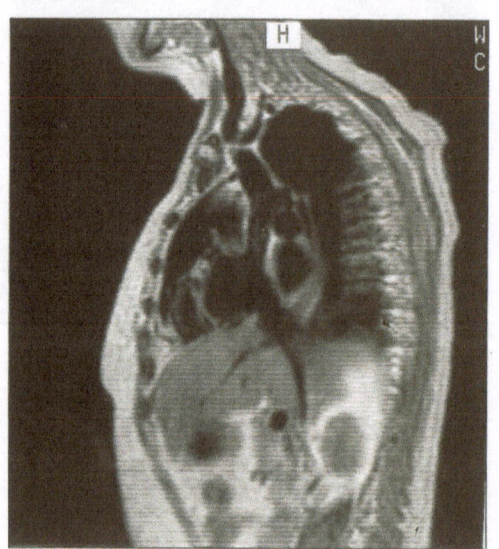

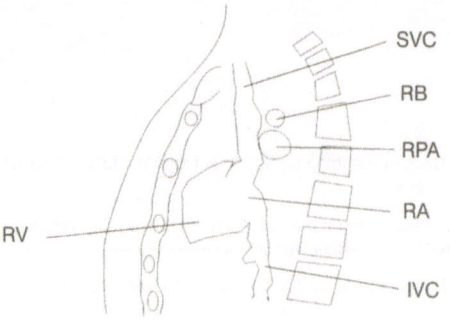

F. 1.22. Programming of a sagittal spin echo sequence on an axial localizing plane.

F. 1.23. Sagittal plane at the level of the vena cava. IVC: inferior vena cava; RA: right atrium; RB: right bronchus; RPA: right pulmonary artery; SVC: superior vena cava.

F. 1.24. Sagittal plane at the level of pulmonary artery. MPA: main pulmonary artery; LV: left ventricle; RVOT: right ventricular outflow tract.

F. 1.25. Sagittal plane at the aortic arch. DAo: descending aorta; IV: innominate vein; LA: left atrium; LSA: left subclavian artery; RA: right atrium; RPA: right pulmonary artery; RV: right ventricle.

F. 1.26. Sagittal plane at the aortic root level. AAo: ascending aorta; IV: innominate vein; LA: left atrium; RPA: right pulmonary artery; RV: right ventricle.

F. 1.27. Sagittal ventricular plane. LV: left ventricle; RV: right ventricle.

FIGURE 1.25

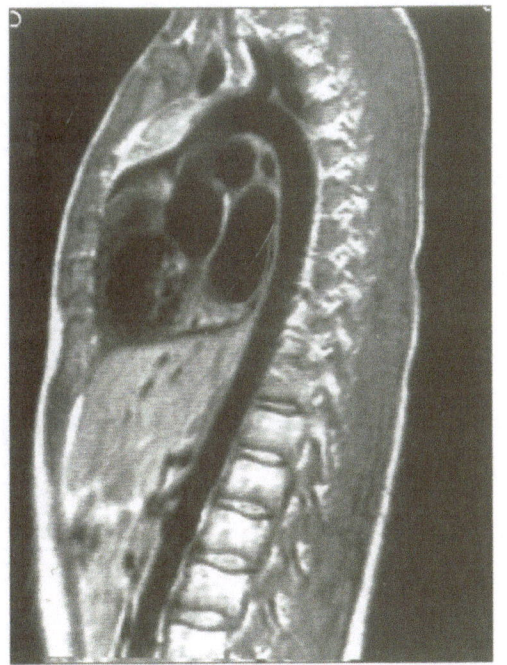

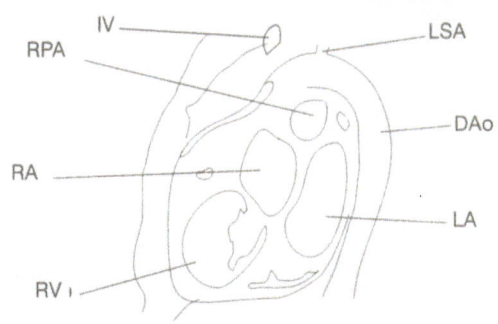

FIGURE 1.26

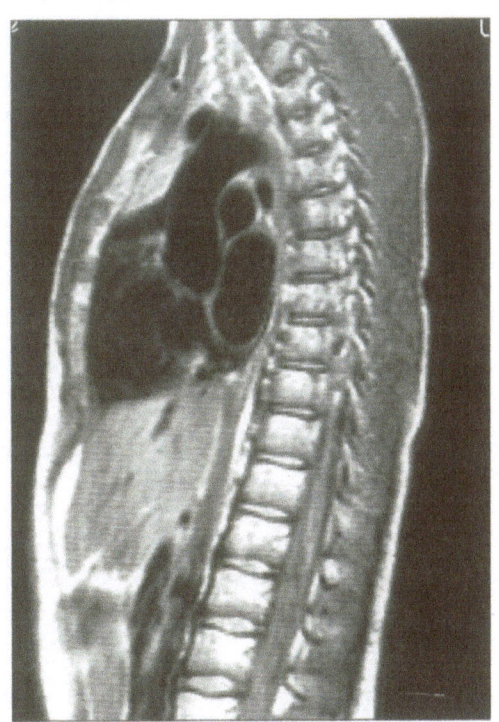

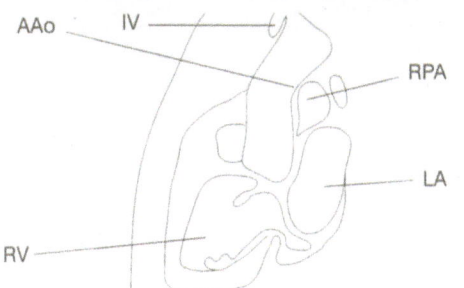

FIGURE 1.27

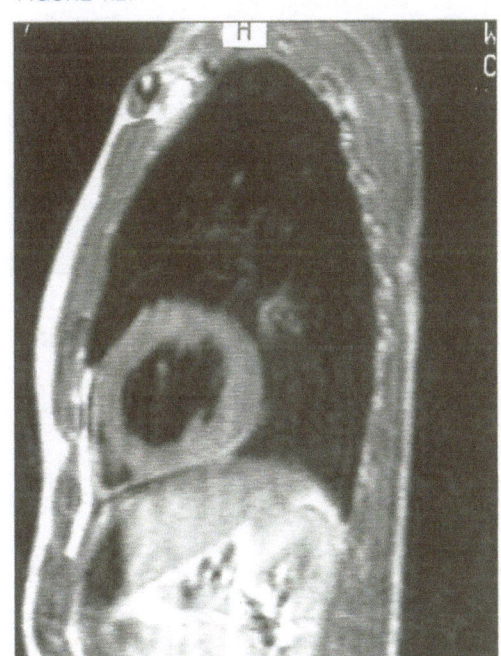

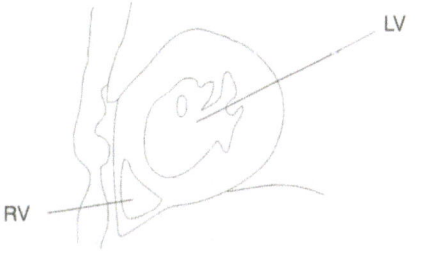

FIGURE 1.28

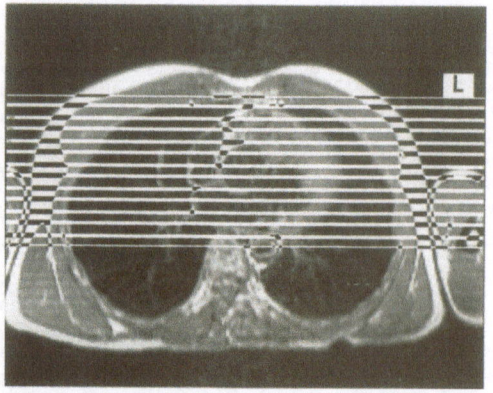

FIGURE 1.29

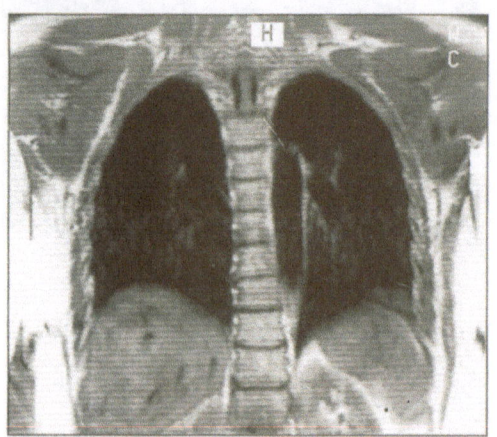

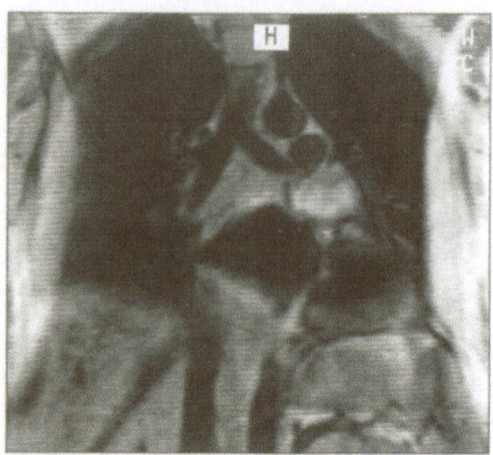

FIGURE 1.30

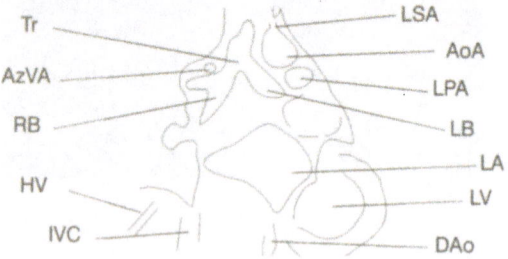

FIGURE 1.31

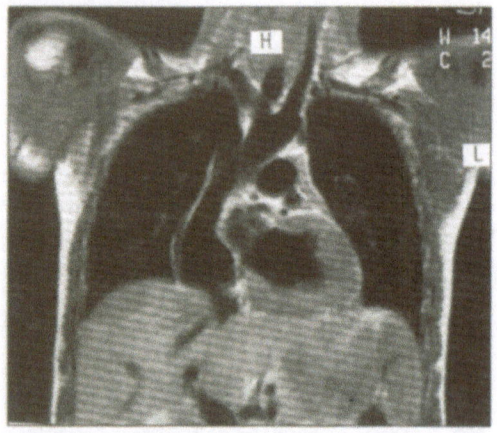

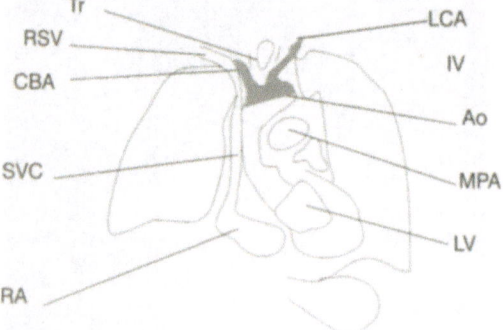

F. 1.28. Programming of a coronal spin-echo sequence superimposed on an axial reference localizing plane.

F. 1.29. Coronal plane on the descending aorta. DAo: descending aorta.

F. 1.30. Coronal plane at the tracheal level. AoA: aortic arch; AzVA: azygous vein arch; DAo: descending aorta; IVC: inferior vena cava; HV: hepatic vein; LA: left atrium; LB: left bronchus; LPA: left pulmonary artery; LSA: left subclavian artery; LV: left ventricle; RB: right bronchus; Tr: trachea.

Coronal plane at the left venticular outflow tract. Ao: aorta; CBA: common brachiocephalic artery; IV: innominate vein; LCA: left carotid artery; LV: left ventricle; MPA: main pulmonary artery; RA: right atrium; RSV: right subclavian vein; SVC: superior vena cava; Tr: trachea.

FIGURE 1.32

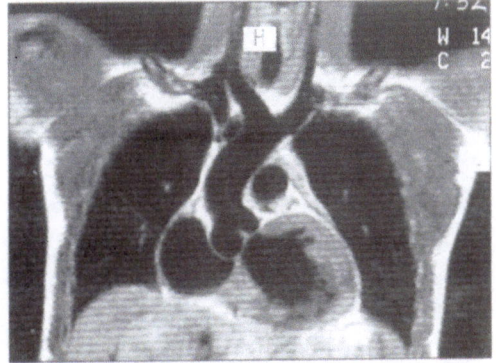

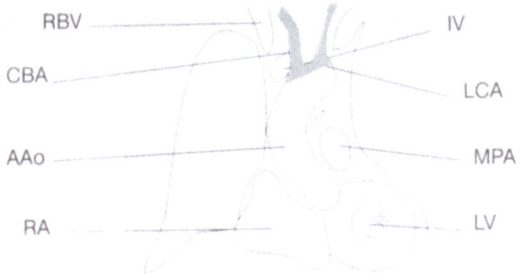

RBV — IV
CBA — LCA
AAo — MPA
RA — LV

FIGURE 1.34

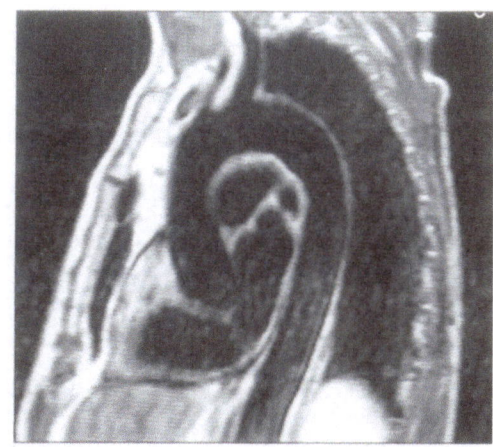

CBA — LCA
Ao
RPA
RB
LA
RA

FIGURE 1.33

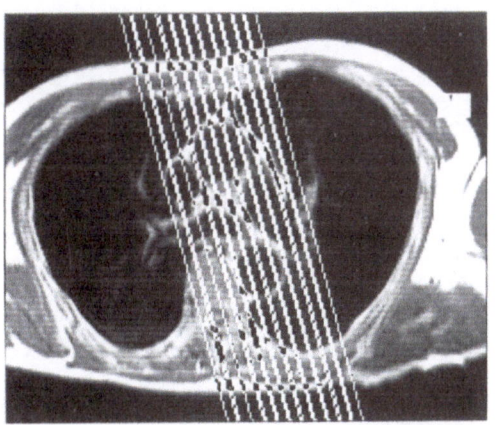

FIGURE 1.35

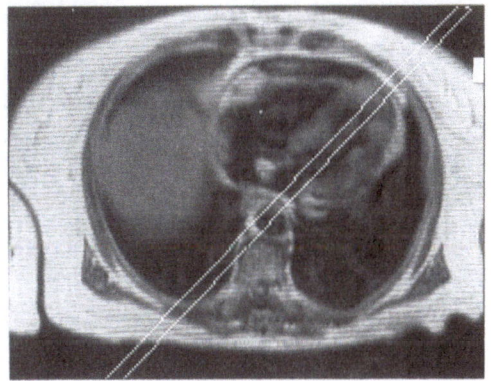

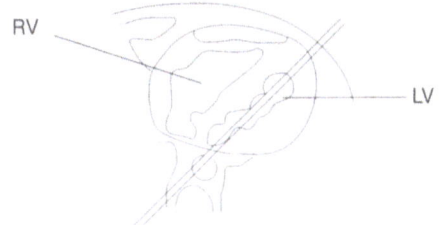

RV — LV

F. 1.32. Coronal plane on the ascending aorta. AAo: ascending aorta; CBA: common brachiocephalic artery; IV: innominate vein; LCA: left carotid artery; LV: left ventricle; MPA: main pulmonary artery; RA: right atrium; RBV: right brachiocephalic vein.

F. 1.33. Programming of a sagittal oblique spin echo sequence, oriented on the plane of the thoracic aorta superimposed on an axial reference localizing plane.

F. 1.34. Sagittal oblique plane of the thoracic aorta. Ao: aorta; CBA: common brachiocephalic artery; LA: left atrium; LCA: left carotid artery; RA: right atrium; RB: right bronchus; RPA: right pulmonary artery.

F. 1.35. Programming of a sagittal oblique slice oriented along the longitudinal axis of the left ventricle superimposed on an axial plane in which the location of the apex and the base of the ventricle are taken as references. LV: left ventricle; RV: right ventricle.

FIGURE 1.36

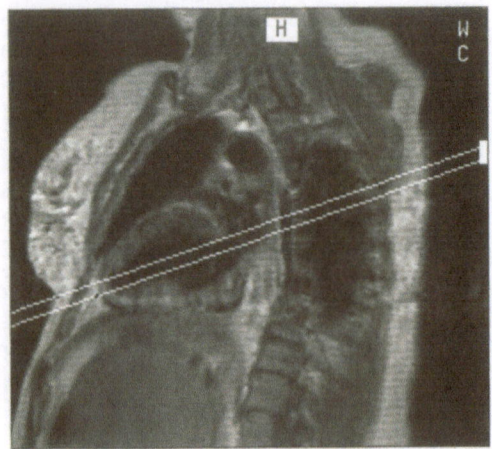

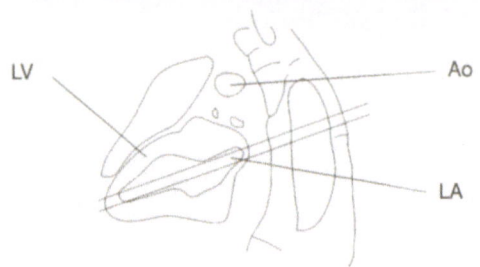

FIGURE 1.38

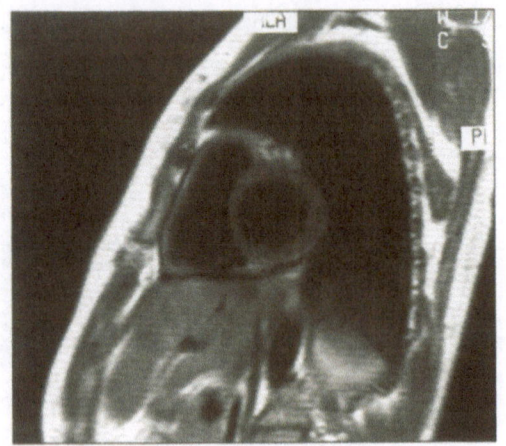

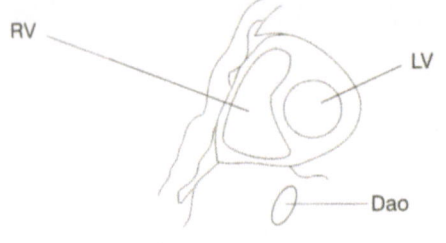

FIGURE 1.37

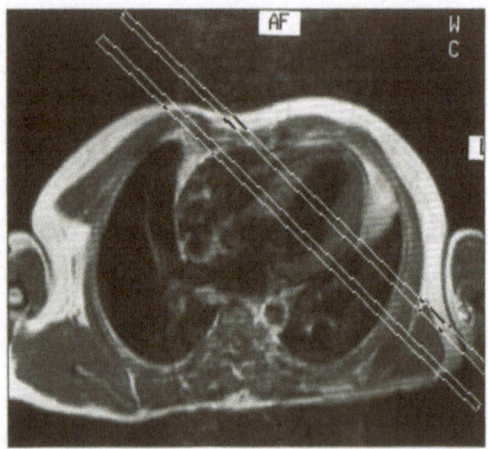

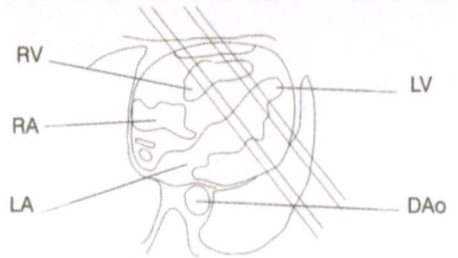

F. 1.36. Sagittal oblique plane of the left ventricle ("2 chambers") obtained with the orientation shown in the previous figure. The programming of a new orthogonal oblique plane is shown also orientated along the longitudinal axis of the left ventricle. Ao: aorta; LA: left atrium; LV: left ventricle.

F. 1.37. Oblique plane along the longitudinal axis of the left ventricle obtained from the programming of the previous figure known as "4 chambers." Programming of two slices of a new oblique sequence oriented on the transversal ventricular plane is shown. DAo: descending aorta; LA: left atrium; LV: left ventricle; RA: right atrium; RV: right ventricle.

F. 1.38. Transverse plane of the left ventricle obtained with the programming of the previous figure. DAo: descending aorta; LV: left ventricle; RV: right ventricle. DAo: descending aorta.

3. Herfkens RJ, Higgins CB, Hricak H, et al. Nuclear magnetic resonance imaging of cardiovascular system: normal and pathological findings. Radiology 1983; 147: 749–59.

4. Higgins CB, Caputo GR. Role of MR imaging in acquired and congenital cardiovascular disease. Am J Röentgenol 1993; 161: 13–22.

5. Pons Lladó G, Carreras F, Gumá JR, et al. Aplicaciones de la resonancia magnética en cardiología: experiencia inicial en 100 casos. Rev Esp Cardiol 1994; 47 (Suppl. 4): 156–65.

6. The clinical role of magnetic resonance in cardiovascular disease. Task Force of the European Society of Cardiology, in collaboration with the Association of European Paediatric Cardiologists. Eur Heart J 1998; 19: 19–39.

7. Budinger TF, Berson A, McVeigh E, et al. Cardiac MR imaging: Report of a Working Group Sponsored by the National Heart, Lung, and Blood Institute. Radiology 1998; 208: 573–6.

8. Hendrick RE, Raff U. Image contrast and noise. In: Stark DD, Bradley WB, ed. Magnetic resonance imaging. St Louis: Mosby-Year Book; 1992: 109–44.

9. von Schulthess GK, Fisher M, Crooks LE, Higgins CB. Gated MR Imaging of the heart: intracardiac signals in patients and healthy subjects. Radiology 1985; 156: 125–32.

10. Sechtem U, Pflugfelder PW, White RD, et al. Cine MR imaging: potential for the evaluation of cardiovascular function. Am J Röentgenol 1987; 148: 239–46.

11. Pettigrew RI. Cardiovascular imaging techniques. In: Stark DD, Bradley WB, ed. Magnetic resonance imaging. St Louis: Mosby-Year Book; 1992: 1605–51.

12. Schwitter J, Sakuma H, Saeed M, Wendland MF, Higgins CB. Very fast cardiac imaging. Magn Reson Imaging Clin North Am 1996; 4: 419–32.

13. Bluemke DA, Boxerman JL, Atalar E, McVeigh ER. Segment K-space cine breath-hold cardiovascular MR imaging: Part 1. Principles and technique. Am J Röentgenol 1997; 169; 395–400.

14. McVeigh ER, Zerhouni EA. Noninvasive measurement of transmural gradients in myocardial strain with MR imaging. Radiology 1991; 180: 677–83.

15. Rebergen S, van der Wall EE, Doornbos J, de Roos A. Magnetic resonance measurement of velocity and flow: technique, validation and cardiovascular applications. Am Heart J 1993; 126: 1439–56.

16. Edelman RR. MR angiography: present and future. Am J Röentgenol 1993; 161: 1–11.

17. Bottomley PA. MR spectroscopy of the heart: the status and the challenges. Radiology 1994; 191: 593–612.

18. Wetter DR, McKinnon GC, Debatin JF, von Schulthess GK. Cardiac echo-planar MR imaging: comparison of single- and multiple shot techniques. Radiology 1995; 194: 765–70.

19. Shellock FG, Morisoli S, Kanal E. MR procedures and biomedical implants, materials, and devices: 1993 update. Radiology 1993; 189: 587–99.

Ventricular morphology and function: study of cardiomyopathies

2

G. PONS-LLADÓ

2.1 Morphological Study of Heart Chambers

a. Left ventricle

The high resolution of magnetic resonance using the spin echo technique allows the acquisition of images of the left ventricle on which it is possible to determine the wall thickness and the chamber diameters. This is due to both the notable spontaneous contrast between the myocardium and the intracavitary flow without the need for contrast agents as well as the possibility it offers of obtaining planes on any orientation. In order to take standard and reproducible measurements, it is important to follow an acquisition strategy which enables a ventricular slice to be obtained on a longitudinal true anatomical plane and during the diastolic phase of the cardiac cycle. Since the long ventricular axis is not generally aligned within any of the natural planes which are systematically used in MRI (axial, coronal and sagittal), it will be necessary to perform a series of angulations: first, it is recommended that an estimate of the orientation of the base and the apex of the left ventricle be taken on one of the axial planes (Figure 2.1); on this plane we will plan a single slice, synchronized with the R wave of the electrocardiogram, that will give an oblique sagittal image which will depict the ventricle along its long axis, including the anterior wall, the ventricular apex and the inferior wall (Figure 2.2). Although this plane already includes the long axis of the left ventricle, a certain amount of artifacts frequently blur the contour of the inferior wall due to movements of the diaphram that is adjacent to it. Therefore, a third sequence is recommended, once again aligning the slice along an imaginary line that includes the apex and the mid point of the mitral plane. This will give us a new longitudinal plane of the left ventricle orthogonal to the previous one, along with the septal and lateral free wall, including the right ventricle and both atria, similar to the echocardiographic four-chamber plane (Figure 2.3). With this slice we can determine the thickness of the left ventricular wall and its transverse diameter. Obviously, these measurements will show good correlation with the corresponding ones obtained by echocardiography[1].

In a good deal of heart diseases, a complete morphological study of the left ventricle must include a determination of the left ventricular mass (LVM). M-mode echocardiography is the most widely used technique[2], although it has limitations, particularly those derived from the diverse geometric assumptions involved in the calculation formula. In spite of the fact that two-dimensional echocardiography (2DE) has theoretical advantages over the M-mode technique, such as its tomographic nature, which would permit more exact determinations of the LVM[3], technical limitations in 2DE studies due to the echographic window and difficulties in recognizing ventricular endocardial and epicardial borders in still images make this method not superior to the M-mode in practice[4].

The advantages of MRI in the determination of LVM reside in its excellent resolution, the absence of image interference due to the intervention of other thoracic structures and the possibility of obtaining left ventricular slices in their full extension and with any orientation. The most common method, which demonstrated in initial studies an extraordinary degree of accuracy with anatomical correlations[5] in experimental animals as well as with isolated human hearts[6], is based on the acquisition of multiple transverse slices of the left ventricle on a plane longitudinal to the ventricle (Figure 2.4) by using spin echo sequences (Figure 2.5A,B). It is generally possible to include the entire extension of the ventricle with 8–10 slices each with a thickness of 8–10 mm. The calculation is made by determining the area of the endocardial and epicardial contours of the left ventricle (Figure 2.6), the difference corresponding to the myocardial area in this section, the volume of which is easily obtained, since the thickness of the slice is determined by the operator. The application of Simpson's rule, by means of the sum of the volume of all the slices studied in this way, results in the total volume of the left ventricular myocardium, which, if multiplied by the density of the myocardial tissue (1.05), will correspond to the LVM in grams. This can be done without the need to apply complex geometric formulas.

One aspect that could constitute a limitation of this method of calculating the LVM is the fact that each one of the transverse sections corresponds to a different phase of the cardiac cycle as the slices are obtained in a single sequence, whether they are obtained by spin echo or gradient echo. This means that we will include in the final calculation sections obtained in the systolic interval together with others in diastole, unless we program as many sequences as slices and obtain images of each section in systole as well as in diastole and then select the diastolic ones for calculation uniformity. Depending upon the number of slices needed to include the entire ventricle, this would increase the examination time by a factor of 8 to 10. Nevertheless, comparative experimental studies of these two techniques in animals[7] and humans[8] have shown an excellent correlation with minimal variability between both of them.

The new modalities of MRI that permit the acquisition of images with very short acquisition times (segmented k-space and echo planar) will undoubtably facilitate the technical aspects of LVM calculation[9], even though the measurement strategy (sum of contiguous sections of the left ventricle) is not modified (Figure 2.7)[10].

One alternative provided by the techniques of rapid acquisition, together with the unlimited possibilities of MRI angulation, is the simplification of LVM calculation by obtaining the measure on a single image of the left ventricle on one of its longitudinal planes (Figure 2.8). Nevertheless, in spite of its extreme rapidity in this case, LVM determination is based in this case on the application of the same geometric formulas that are used in 2DE[3]. The method is, therefore, indirect in comparison with the technique of multiple transverse slices.

In our own experience[11], the determination of LVM using the MRI technique of spin echo transverse slices demonstrates good correlation with echocardiographic calculations, except in those patients with asymmetrical forms of hypertrophy, where it can be assumed that echocardiographic measurement is inadequate. Likewise, the comparison between the previously mentioned method of transverse slices and that of LVM calculation on a longitudinal slice obtained with a rapid sequence of segmented-k-space demonstrates an excellent correlation

28

FIGURE 2.1

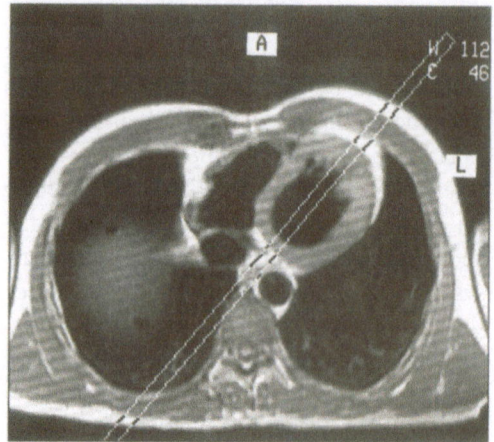

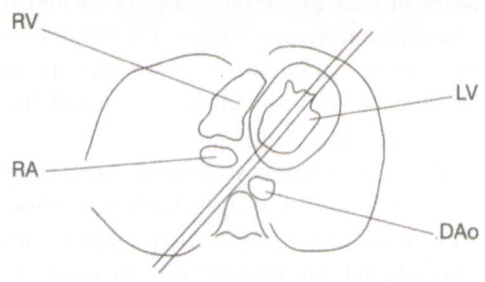

FIGURE 2.3

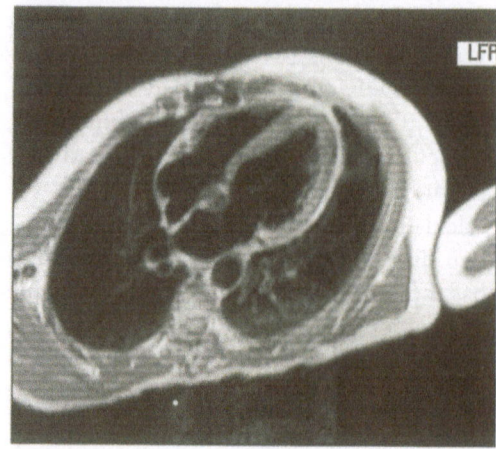

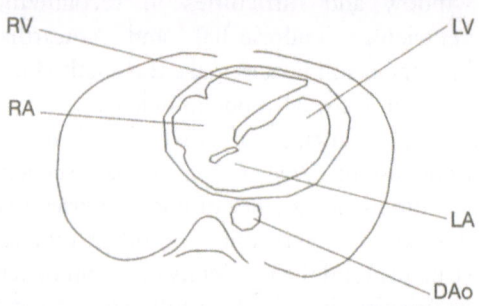

FIGURE 2.2

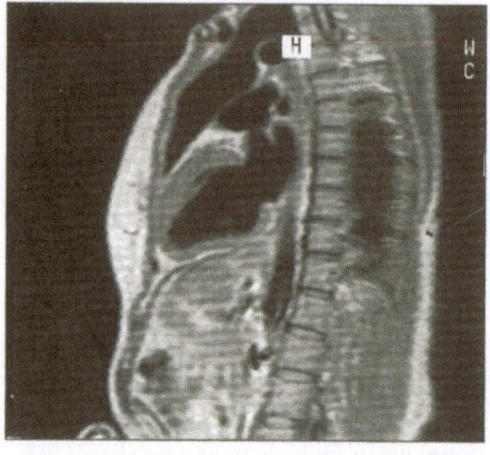

FIGURE 2.4

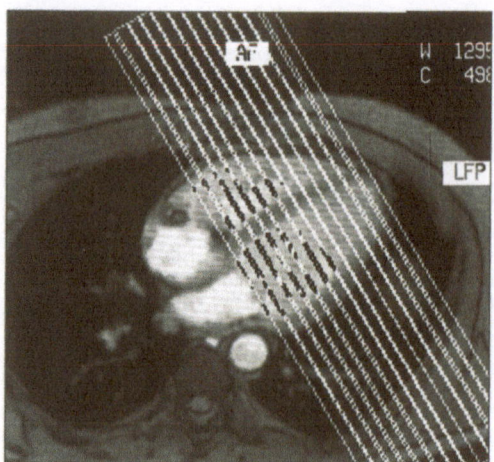

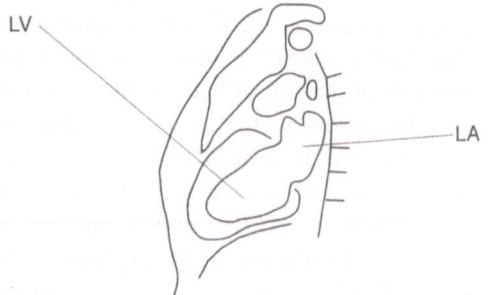

F. 2.1.   Programming of an oblique sagittal slice oriented along the longitudinal axis of the left ventricle over an axial plane in which the localization of the apex and the base of the ventricle are taken as references. DAo: descending aorta; LV: left ventricle; RA: right atrium; RV: right ventricle.

F. 2.2.   Oblique sagittal plane of the left ventricle ("2 chambers") obtained with the orientation shown in Figure 2.1. LA: left atrium; LV: left ventricle.

F. 2.3.   Plane of "4 chambers" of the heart in which the left ventricle is represented on a longitudinal plane orthogonal to that depicted in Figure 2.2. DAo: descending aorta; LA: left atrium; LV: left ventricle; RA: right atrium; RV: right ventricle.

F. 2.4.   Programming of a spin echo sequence superimposed on transverse planes of the left ventricle.

FIGURE 2.5 A and B

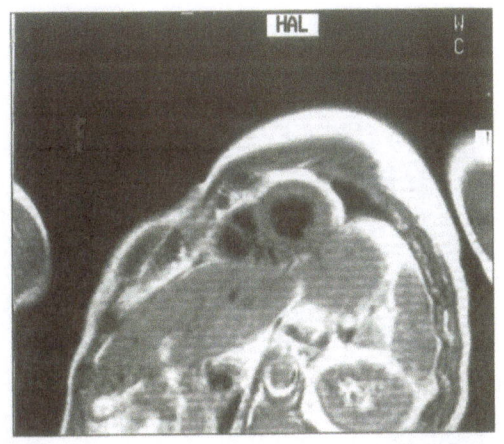 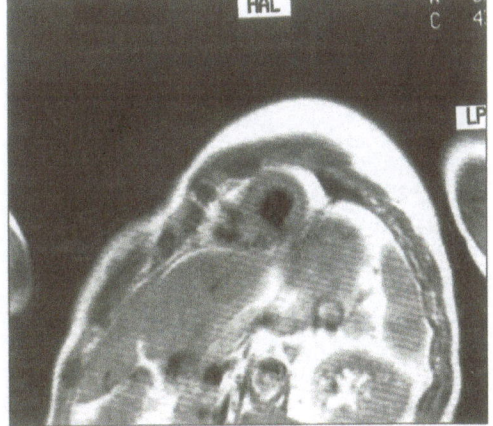

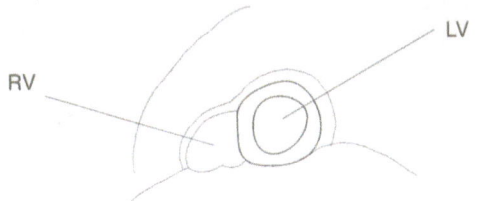 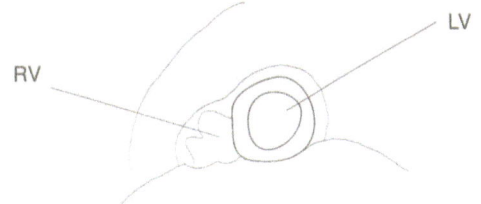

FIGURE 2.6

FIGURE 2.7

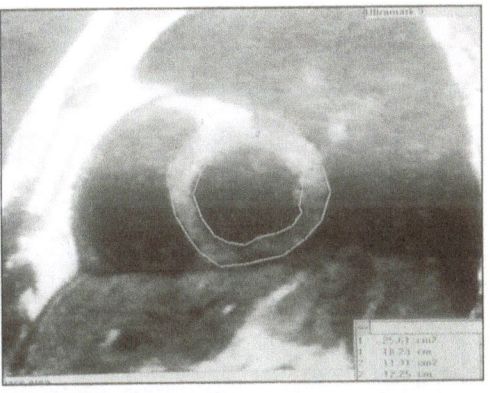 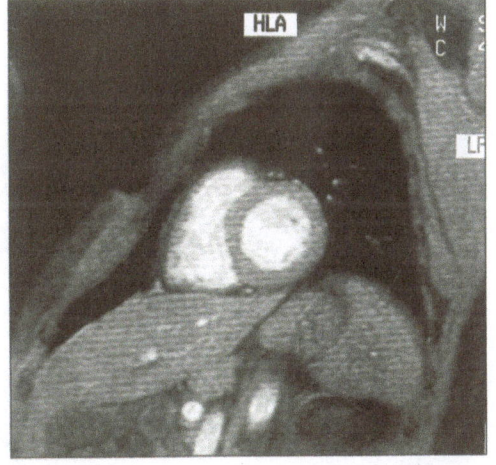

F. 2.5 (A) and (B). Examples of spin echo transverse planes of the left ventricle in two levels of the cavity. LV: left venticle; RV: right ventricle.

F. 2.6. Determination of the endocardial and epicardial areas of a transverse slice of the left ventricle in order to calculate the ventricular mass.

F. 2.7. Transverse plane of the left ventricle obtained with a rapid sequence using segmented-k-space technique.

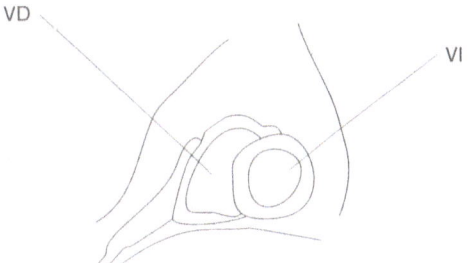

FIGURE 2.8

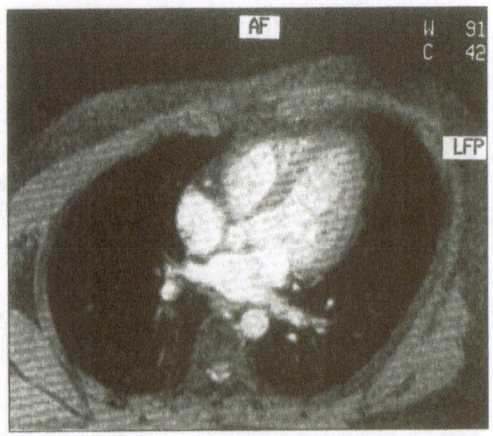

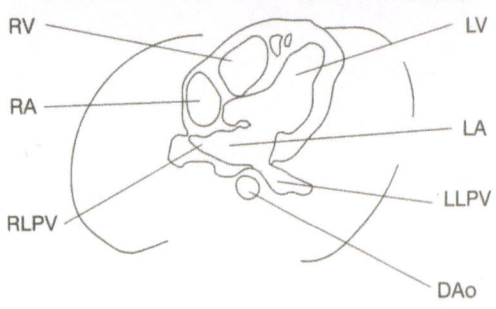

RV
LV
RA
LA
LLPV
RLPV
DAo

FIGURE 2.10

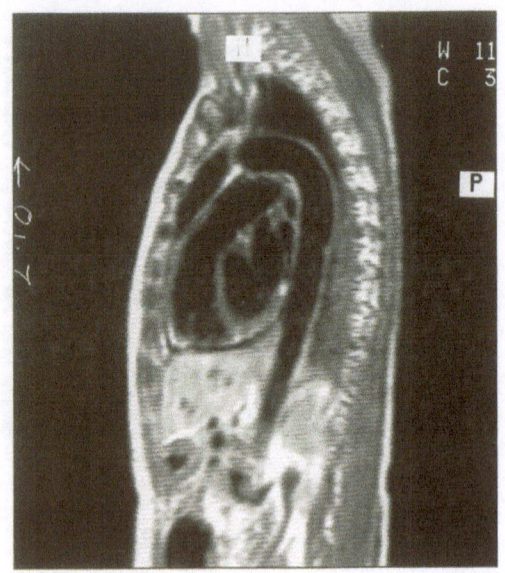

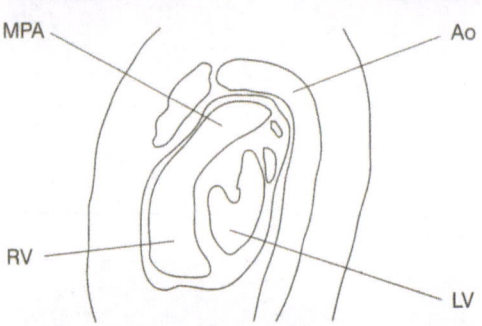

MPA
Ao
RV
LV

FIGURE 2.9 A and B

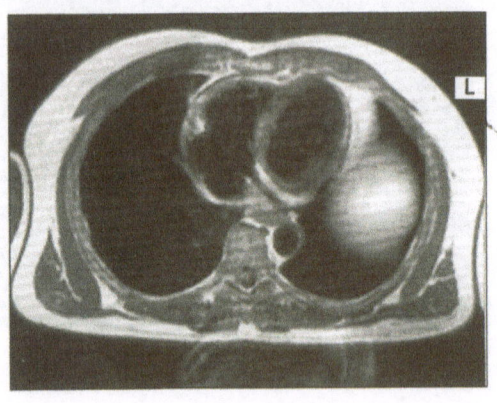

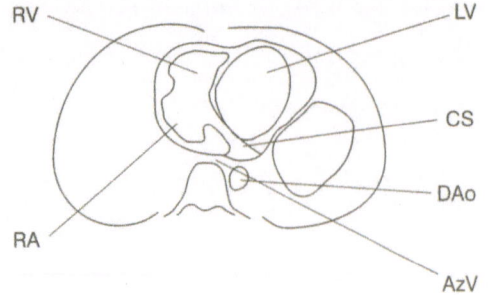

RV
LV
CS
DAo
RA
AzV

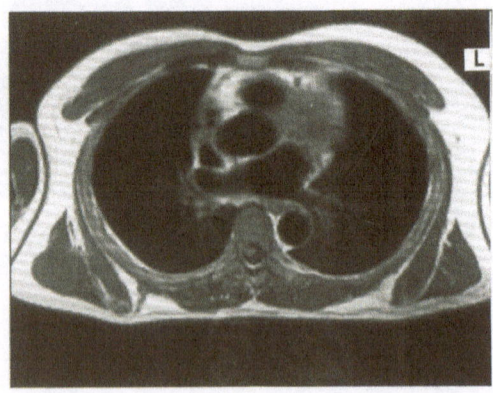

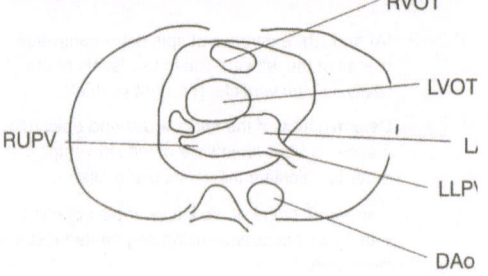

RVOT
LVOT
RUPV
L
LLPV
DAo

between both, and the latter can be considered a valid alternative of simple application for the determination of LVM by MRI. The excellent reproducibility of LVM measurement by MRI should be noted. It is clearly superior to that obtained by echocardiography[12], which has important practical applications in those cases in which a series of determinations of this parameter are required, particularly when the objective is to estimate the possible evolutionary changes of ventricular hypertrophy.

b. Right ventricle

Due to the complex morphology of the right ventricle, it is necessary to consider in its evaluation two anatomical regions: the inflow and outflow chambers. In axial slices the limit between both is determined by the change in configuration of the chamber, from triangular for the inflow chamber, which appears in lower in axial slices, to circular in the outflow chamber, situated above (Figure 2.9A,B). The latter is also easily delimited in sagittal slices (Figure 2.10). Based on these images it is possible to determine the right ventricular wall thickness, which in normal individuals is 3 ± 1 mm, as well as the maximum diameters of the chamber, the normal values being 32 ± 5 mm in the inflow chamber and 26 ± 4 mm in the outflow portion[13]. It is important to point out that the slices which are measured should be necessarily obtained in ventricular diastole, which, with the spin echo technique, requires the use of an acquisition strategy similar to that described for the left ventricle, i.e. sychronization with the R wave of the electrocardiogram.

Although it is theoretically possible to determine also the right ventricular mass using MRI by following the method consisting of summing the contiguous transverse slices, similar to that which was described for the left ventricle[14], the already mentioned particularly complex morphology of the ventricular cavity causes this method to be less reliable than in the case of the left ventricle. Due to the fact, however, that the right ventricular mass is of only relative clinical interest, this procedure is not common practice.

2.2   Ventricular Function

a. Left ventricular function

MRI permits an adequate estimation of the volume of the left ventricular cavity, either by adding the calculation of the volume of each one of the slices in a transverse series that covers the entire extension of the cavity, a strategy similar to the one described for measuring the LVM (Figure 2.5A,B), or by the application of any of the formulas for measuring volume from a longitudinal plane of the ventricle (Figure 2.3)[15]. It must be considered, however, that in order to determine the ventricular ejection fraction, it is necessary to obtain systolic and diastolic volumes. This implies that, when the method of adding partial volumes of contiguous transverse slices is applied, a large number of sequences must be obtained (one for every slice), selecting in each case the end-diastolic and end-systolic ones for the calculation. The process is, thus, very time consuming, although it has been demonstrated that the method is highly accurate[16]. For this reason, it is more suitable to use cine MRI in gradient echo on a longitudinal plane of the ventricle. The image of maximum and minimum ventricular volume is selected (Figure 2.11A,B), and any one of the methods of volume calculation used in E2D is applied (Figure 2.12). Comparative angiographic studies have demonstrated good correlation with this method, particularly if the

---

F. 2.8.   "4-chamber" plane of the heart including the longitudinal plane of the left ventricle obtained with a rapid sequence by segmented k-space technique.; DAo: descending aorta; LA: left atrium; LLPV: left lower pulmonary vein; LV: left ventricle ; RA: right atrium; RLPV: right lower pulmonary vein; RV: right ventricle

F. 2.9.   Determination of the dimensions of the right ventricle in spin echo axial planes. A: ventricular inflow chamber; B: outflow tract. AzV: azygous vein; DAo: descending aorta; CS: coronary sinus; LA: left atrium; LLPV: left lower pulmonary vein; LV: left ventricle; LVOT: left ventricular outflow tract; RA: right atrium; RUPV: right upper pulmonary vein; RV: right ventricle; RVOT: right ventricular outflow tract.

F. 2.10.   Sagittal plane in spin echo on the right ventricular outflow tract. Ao: aorta; LV: left ventricle; MPA: main pulmonary artery; RV: right ventricle.

FIGURE 2.11 A and B

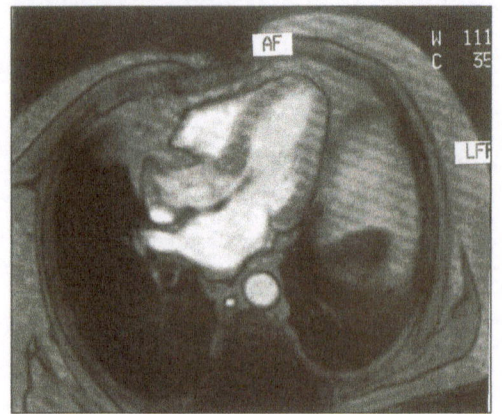

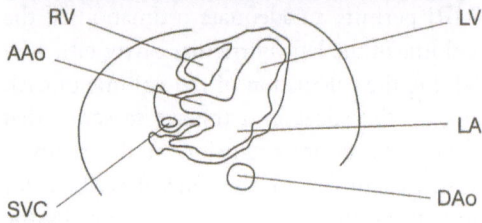

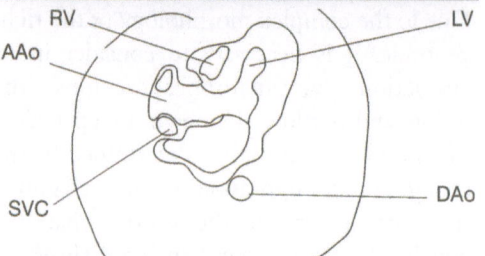

FIGURE 2.12

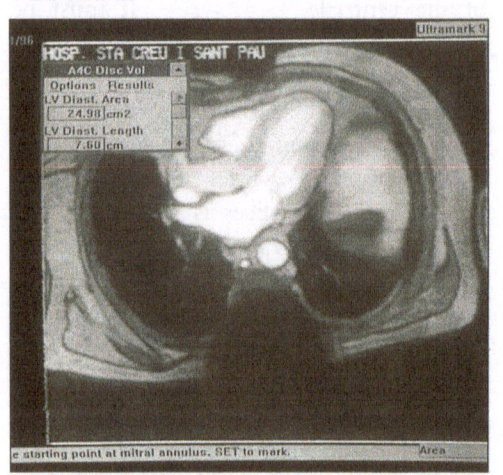

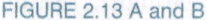

FIGURE 2.13 A and B

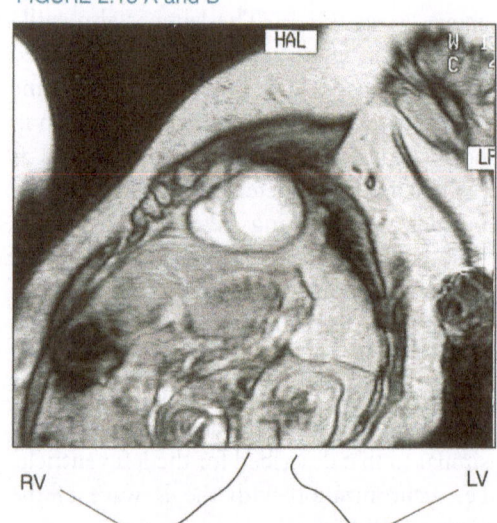

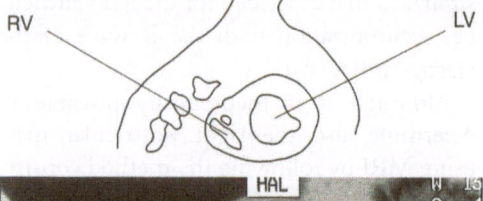

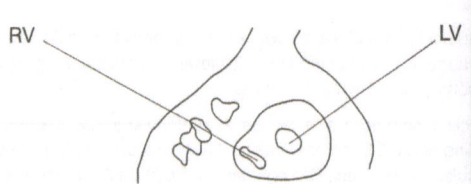

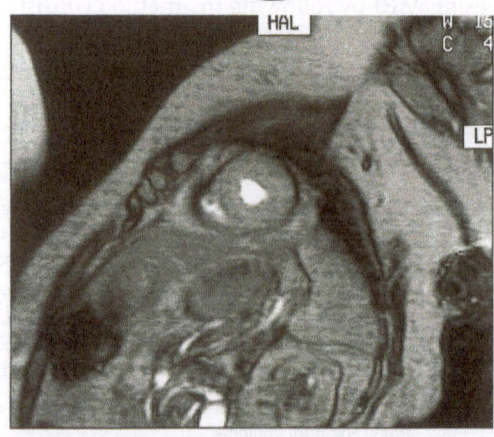

calculation is applied by averaging the volumes obtained along two longitudinal orthogonal slices of the left ventricle[17]. It must be pointed out, nevertheless, that in the case of an important deformation of the ventricular contour, such as in a parietal aneurysm, the simplification of assuming a geometric form for the calculation of the cavity volumes is not appropriate. The application of the method of summation of partial volumes of transverse contiguous slices is then necessary in these cases[18].

Of particular interest in patients with ischemic heart disease is the assessment of the regional left ventricular function. MRI can be used to this end by means of one or a series of cine MRI sequences in gradient echo oriented transverse to the left ventricle. It is possible to determine the diastolic thickness of each segment as well as its systolic thickness (Figure 2.13A,B), parameters which have been demonstrated to be of utility in the estimation of regional myocardial ischemic damage, and even of its potential viability[19]. The tedious large number of measurements on the digitized images that are required for these calculations when practiced manually may be considerably alleviated by the application of semiautomated contour detection algorithms[20].

b. Right ventricular function

It is not possible to assume simple geometric forms for the measurement of the right ventricular volume due to its special morphology, as is the case of the left ventricle when a dyskinetic area or aneurysm is present. Under these conditions the calculation of volumes and the ejection fraction requires the use of Simpson's rule, with the sum of the cavity areas obtained by contiguous, multiple slices of the ventricle in telediastole and telesystole. This method is considered to be the most exact, but its implementation requires considerable time, which makes it of little practical use in clinical practice, although it is the method of reference for research studies[21].

2.3 Cardiomyopathies

a. Dilated cardiomyopathy

Although the diagnosis of dilated cardiomyopathy by echocardiography does not, in general, present difficulties and, therefore, there is no definite indication for MRI in the diagnosis of cardiomyopathy, its use can, on the other hand, be considered for follow-up studies of left ventricular volume and function due to its high reproducibiliy, which is of particular interest in studies of pharmacological intervention[22].

b. Hypertrophic cardiomyopathy

The diagnostic role of echocardiography in this area is not disputed, since, due to its application, it has been possible not only to detect its presence[23] but also to determine the extension of ventricular hypertrophy[24]. The limitations, nevertheless, of ultrasound in certain patients are known[25]. They are particularly problematic in hypertrophic cardiomyopathy, where the process may be confined to specific regions of the left ventricle, which may be eventually not visualized by ultrasound[26]. MRI offers then a valid alternative for the systematic study of wall thickness of the left ventricle in hypertrophic cardiomyopathy[27,28], especially in uncommon forms such as where hypertrophy is limited to the apical region[29].

The study method is the same that was described for the analysis of left ventricular morphology. Using the spin echo technique, longitudinal planes of the left ventricle are obtained (Figure 2.14), as well as transverse planes (Figure 2.15), which permit an adequate estimation of the degree and extension of the hypertrophic process[30]. The importance of obtaining planes in the diastolic phase of the

F. 2.11. **Diastolic (A) and systolic (B) images of a cine MRI sequence in gradient echo oriented on a longitudinal plane of the left ventricle. AAo: ascending aorta; DAo: descending aorta; LA: left atrium; LV: left ventricle ; RV: right ventricle; SVC: superior vena cava.**

F. 2.12. **Determination of the left ventricular chamber volume using a conventional planimetry method.**

F. 2.13. **Diastolic (A) and systolic (B) images of a cine MRI sequence in gradient echo oriented on a transverse plane of the left ventricle.**

FIGURE 2.14

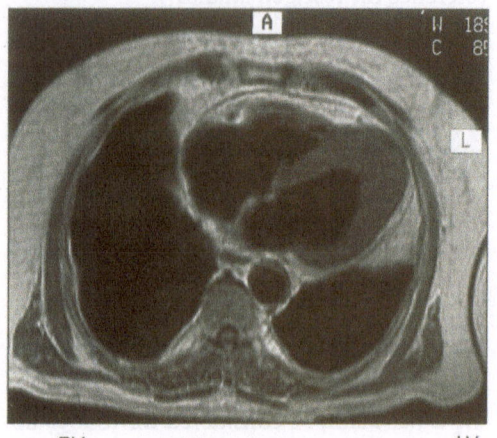

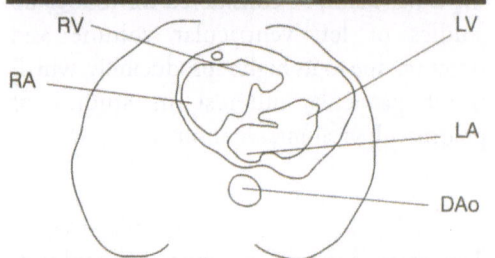

FIGURE 2.15

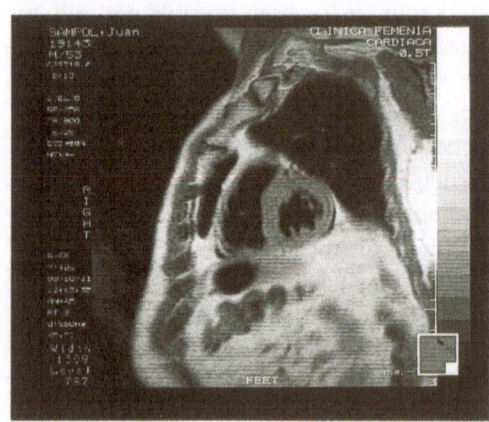

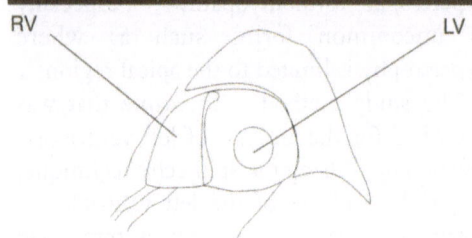

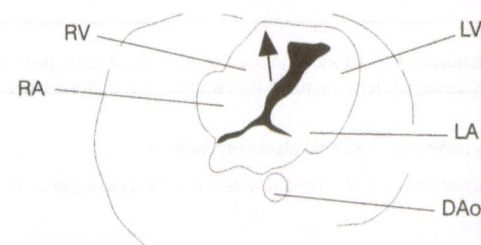

FIGURE 2.16

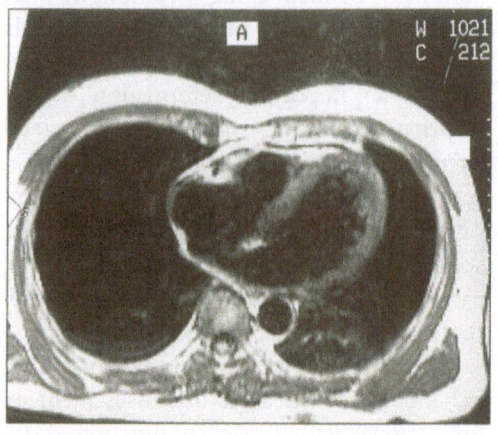

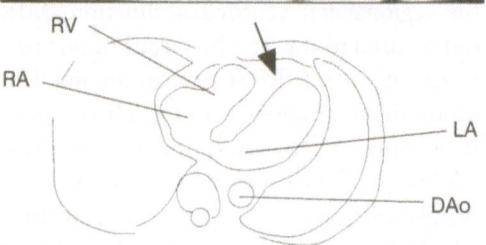

FIGURE 2.17 A and B

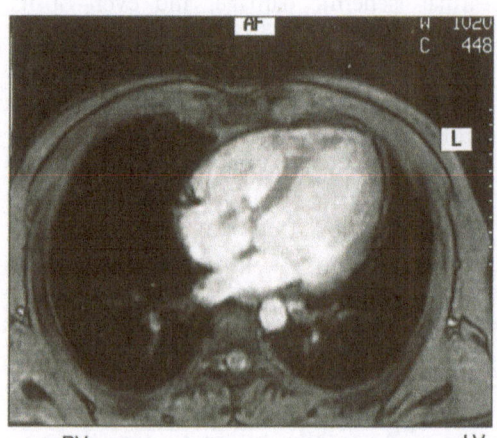

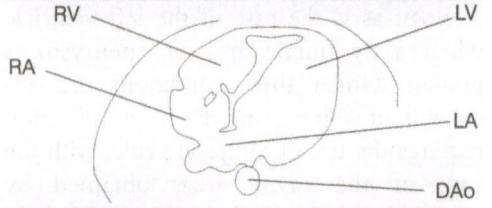

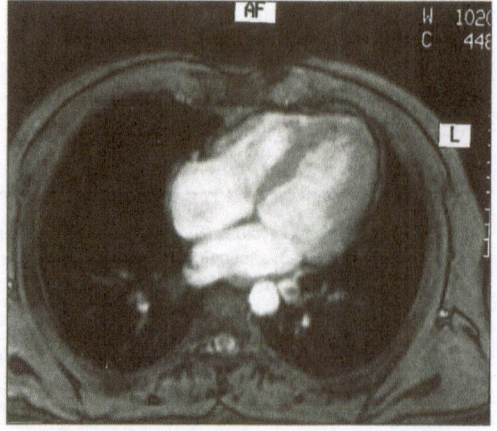

cardiac cycle in order to carry out a reproducible measurement of the parietal thickness must be emphasized. For the purposes of a follow-up study it is also possible to determine the ventricular mass by the method described above, which also yields a high degree of reproducibility[31].

c. Restrictive cardiomyopathy

There are no distinctive morphological features of restrictive cardiomyopathy using MRI, which also holds true for other diagnostic methods, although the possibility of evaluating the differences between signal intensity of the myocardium in cases of amyloid infiltration and signal intensity in cases of simple hypertrophy has been suggested[32].

MRI is useful, on the other hand, in the differential diagnosis between restrictive cardiomyopathy and constrictive pericarditis[33], an arduous problem in practice, which is possible in this case due to the high resolution of the technique for detecting pericardial thickening, even of a mild degree, which is indicative of constriction, as will be discussed in the chapter devoted to constrictive pericarditis.

d. Arrhythmogenic dysplasia of the right ventricle

This genetically transmitted condition is defined by the presence of arrhythmias originating in the right ventricle with evidence of contractile dysfunction of the cavity, whether global or segmental. Until recently, the diagnosis was based on a ventricular angiography and an endomyocardial biopsy, which frequently show focal points of intramyocardial fat infiltration[34]. MRI studies have demonstrated the utility of

the technique in the diagnosis of dysplasia by identifying fat infiltration in the right ventricular myocardium (Figure 2.16)[35]. Although a very specific finding, it is only present in a proportion of cases[36]. Alternatively, the technique permits the identification of focal wall thinning or bulges and of segmental right ventricular contraction abnormalities that are of diagnostic value (Figure 2.17A,B) and that can be also found in patients in whom the diagnostic criteria of arrhythmogenic dysplasia are not fulfilled but who present with frequent apparently unexplained premature contractions originating in the right ventricle[37].

References

1. Kaul S, Wismer GL, Brady TJ, et al. Measurement of normal left heart dimensions using optimally oriented MR images. Am J Röentgenol 1986; 146: 75–9.

2. Devereux RB, Alonso DR, Lutas EM, et al. Echocardiographic assessment of left ventricular hypertrophy: comparison to necropsy findings. Am J Cardiol 1986; 57: 450–8.

3. Schiller NB, Skiodebrand C, Schiller E, et al. In vivo assessment of left ventricular mass by two-dimensional echocardiography. Circulation 1983; 68: 210–5.

4. Devereux RB. Detection of left ventricular hypertrophy by M-mode echocardiography: anatomic validation, standardization, and comparison to other methods. Hypertension 1987; 9 (Suppl. II): II-19–II-26.

5. Florentine MS, Grosskreutz CL, Chang W, et al. Measurement of left ventricular mass in vivo using gated nuclear magnetic resonance imaging. J Am Coll Cardiol 1986; 8: 107–12.

F. 2.14. "4 chamber" plane of the heart using the spin echo technique in a case of hypertrophic cardiomyopathy that affects the apical portion of the left ventricle. Note the relative normal thickness of the basal segments of the ventricular wall. DAo: descending aorta; LA: left atrium; LV: left ventricle; RA: right atrium; RV: right ventricle.

F. 2.15. Transverse plane of the left ventricle using the spin echo technique in a case of hypertrophic cardiomyopathy involving the interventricular septum. Note the normal thickness of the left ventricular free wall and, also, of the right ventricular wall. LV: left ventricle; RV: right ventricle.

F. 2.16. Axial plane on spin echo in a case of arrhythmogenic dysplasia of the right ventricle. There is fat infiltration in the free anterior wall of the chamber which is identifiable due to the high signal intensity of the adipose tissue (arrow): compare with the intensity of the normal intermediate signal of the left ventricular wall. DAo: descending aorta; LA: left atrium; LV: left ventricle; RA: right atrium; RV: right ventricle.

F. 2.17. Diastolic (A) and systolic (B) images of a cine MRI sequence using the gradient echo technique in a case of arrhythmogenic dysplasia. Observe the region of segmental dysfunction of the right ventricular wall with systolic bulging (arrow in B). DAo: descending aorta; LA: left atrium; LV: left ventricle; RA: right atrium; RV: right ventricle.

6. Katz J, Milliken MC, Stray-Gundersen J, et al. Estimation of human myocardial mass with MR imaging. Radiology 1988; 169: 495–8.

7. Shapiro EP, Rogers WJ, Beyar R, et al. Determination of left ventricular mass by magnetic resonance imaging in hearts deformed by acute infarction. Circulation 1989; 79: 706–11.

8. Aurigemma G, Davidoff A, Silver K, Boehmer J, Serio A, Pattison N. Left ventricular mass quantitation using single-phase cardiac magnetic resonance imaging. Am J Cardiol 1992; 70: 259–62.

9. Sakuma H, Fugita N, Foo TK, et al. Evaluation of left ventricular volume and mass with breath-hold cine MR imaging. Radiology 1993; 188: 377–80.

10. McDonald KM, Parrish T, Wennberg P, et al. Rapid, accurate and simultaneous noninvasive assessment of right and left ventricular mass with nuclear magnetic resonance imaging using the snapshot gradient method. J Am Coll Cardiol 1992; 19: 1601–7.

11. Pons-Lladó G, Carreras F, Borrás X, Llauger J, Palmer J, Bayés de Luna A. Left ventricular mass by echocardiography and magnetic resonance (abstract). J Cardiovasc Magn Reson 1999; 1: 91–2.

12. Germain P, Roul G, Kastler B, Mossard JM, Bareiss P, Sacrez A. Inter-study variability in left ventricular mass measurement. Comparison between M-mode echography and MRI. Eur Heart J 1992; 13: 1011–9.

13. Markievicz W, Sechtem U, Higgins CB. Evaluation of the right ventricle by magnetic resonance imaging. Am Heart J 1987; 113: 8–15.

14. Katz J, Whang J, Boxt LM, Barst RJ. Estimation of right ventricular mass in normal subjects and in patients with primary pulmonary hypertension by nuclear magnetic resonance imaging. J Am Coll Cardiol 1993; 21: 1475–81.

15. Underwood SR, Gill CRW, Firmin DN, et al. Left ventricular volume measured rapidly by oblique magnetic resonance imaging. Br Heart J 1988; 60: 188–95.

16. Pattynama PM, Lamb HJ, van der Velde EA, van der Wall EE, de Roos A. Left ventricular measurements with cine and spin-echo MR imaging: a study of reproducibility with variance component analysis. Radiology 1993; 187: 261–8.

17. Cranney GB, Lotan CS, Dean L, Baxley W, Bouchard A, Pohost GM. Left ventricular volume measurement using cardiac axis nuclear magnetic resonance imaging. Validation by calibrated ventricular angiography. Circulation 1990; 82: 154–63.

18. Semelka RC, Tomei E, Wagner S, et al. Interstudy reproducibility of dimensional and functional measurements between cine magnetic resonance studies in the morphologically abnormal left ventricle. Am Heart J 1990; 119: 1367–73.

19. Sechtem U, Sommerhoff BA, Markiewicz W, et al. Regional left ventricular wall thickness by MRI: evaluation in normal subjects and patients with global and regional dysfunction. Am J Cardiol 1987; 59: 145–51.

20. van der Geest RJ, Buller VG, Jansen E, et al. Comparison between manual and semi-automated analysis of left ventricular volume parameters from short-axis MR images. J Comput Assist Tomogr 1997; 21: 756–65.

21. Pattynama PM, Lamb HJ, Van der Welde EA, Van der Geest RJ, Van der Wall EE, de Roos A. Reproducibility of MRI-derived measurements of right ventricular volumes and myocardial mass. Magn Reson Imaging 1995; 13: 53–63.

22. Doherty NE III, Seelos KC, Suzuki J, et al. Application of cine NMR imaging for sequential evaluation of response to angiotensin converting enzyme inhibitor therapy in dilated cardiomyopathy. J Am Coll Cardiol 1992; 19: 1294–302.

23. Maron BJ, Gootdiener JS, Epstein SE. Patterns and significance of distribution of left ventricular hypertrophy: wide-angle, two-dimensional echocardiographic study of 125 patients. Am J Cardiol 1981; 48: 418–28.

24. Candell-Riera J, Alvarez-Auñón A, Balda-Caravedo F, García del Castillo H, Soler-Soler J. Clasificación de la miocardiopatía hipertrófica mediante ecocardiografía bidimensional. Rev Esp Cardiol 1986; 39: 358–63.

25. Geiser EA, Skorton DJ, Conetta DA. Quantification of left ventricular function by two-dimensional echocardiography: consideration of factors restricting image quality. Am Heart J 1982; 103: 905–11.

26. Maron BJ, Spirito P, Chiarella F, Vecchio C. Unusual distribution of left ventricular hypertrophy in obstructive hypertrophic cardiomyopathy: localized posterobasal free wall thickening in two patients. J Am Coll Cardiol 1985; 5: 1474–7.

27. Park JH, Kim YM, Chung JW, Park YB, Han JK, Han MC. MR imaging of hypertrophic cardiomyopathy. Radiology 1992; 185: 441–6.

28. Sardanelli F, Molinari G, Petillo A, et al. MRI in hypertrophic cardiomyopathy: a morphofunctional study. J Comput Assist Tomogr 1993; 17: 862–72.

29. Suzuki J, Watanabe F, Takenaka K, et al. New subtype of apical hypertrophic cardiomyopathy identified with nuclear magnetic resonance imaging as an underlying cause of markedly inverted T waves. J Am Coll Cardiol 1993; 22: 1175–81.

30. Pons-Lladó G, Carreras F, Borrás X, Llauger J, Palmer J, Bayés de Luna A. Comparison of morphologic assessment of hypertrophic cardiomyopathy by magnetic resonance versus echocardiographic imaging. Am J Cardiol 1997; 79: 1651–6.

31. Allison JD, Flickinger FW, Wright JC, et al. Measurement of left ventricular mass in hypertrophic cardiomyopathy using MRI: comparison with echocardiography. Magn Reson Imaging 1993; 11: 329–34.

32. Fattori R, Rocchi G, Celletti R, Bertaccini P, Descovich B, Gavelli G. Differential diagnosis of cardiac amyloidosis and symmetrical hypertrophic cardiomyopathy: morphological features and tissue characterization by MRI. Circulation 1996; 94 (Suppl. I): I-122–3.

33. Masui T, Finck S, Higgins CB. Constrictive pericarditis and restrictive cardiomyopathy: evaluation with MR imaging. Radiology 1992; 182: 369–73.

34. Mc Kenna WJ, Thiene G, Nava A, et al. Diagnosis of arrhythmogenic right ventricular dysplasia/cardiomyopathy. Br Heart J 1994; 71: 215–8.

35. Aufferman W, Withcher T, Breithardt G, Joachimsen K, Peters PE. Arrhythmogenic right ventricular disease: MR imaging vs. angiography. Am J Röentgenol 1993; 161: 549–55.

36. Menghetti L, Basso C, Nava A, Angelini A, Thiene G. Spin-echo nuclear magnetic resonance for tissue characterisation in arrhythmogenic right ventricular cardiomyopathy. Heart 1996; 76: 467–70.

37. Proclemer A, Basadonna PT, Slavich GA, Miani D, Fresco C, Fioretti PM. Cardiac magnetic resonance imaging findings in patients with right ventricular outflow tract premature contractions. Eur Heart J 1997; 18: 2002–10.

Acquired diseases of the aorta

3

G. PONS-LLADÓ

The recent introduction of the cardiac applications of MRI has provided a new and interesting diagnostic tool which has been successfully applied in a wide number of cardiovascular entities. Although its cost-efficiency relation has not been proven in all fields[1], in the specific cases of congenital and acquired aortic diseases, MRI is at present a technique that must be systematically considered. Although the information provided by the method frequently overlaps in some aspects with that obtained by other imaging methods, it has certain advantages over them (Table 3.1). For practical purposes, the following features of MRI can be highlighted: its noninvasive character, the possibility of obtaining planes of the entire aortic length with any orientation without using contrast agents, its excellent image definition and easily-understood presentation format.

3.1 Technical Aspects of the Aortic Study by MRI: Imaging the Normal Aorta

Due to the longitudinal disposition of this vessel in the body, transverse sections can be obtained along the axial planes (perpendicular to the cranio-caudal axis of the body) of the thorax and the abdomen, while along both coronal (frontal) and sagittal (antero-posterior) planes the aorta is represented in longitudinal views. Nevertheless, due to the orientation of the vessel, at least in the normal aorta, oblique sagittal planes are frequently required in order to visualize all its segments in the same image.

Although diverse application modalities of MRI exist, some of them only available on the most advanced systems, the basic equipment found on all commercial equipment is sufficient for an adequate study of the aorta. It should be noted, nevertheless, that in order to obtain images of good resolution it is necessary, in any case, to take ECG-gated sequences.

The spin echo T1-weighted technique provides static images with excellent resolution for the study of aortic morphology, including its caliber and the wall characteristics along its entire course (Figures 3.1 A-E). As is known,

Table 3.1 Comparative diagnostic usefulness of the different diagnostic techniques in the study of aortic disease

	Plain radiography	Contrast angiography	CAT scanner	Echo (external)	Echo (esophageal)	MRI
Noninvasive character	+	–	+	++	–	++
Field of vision	+	+	++	+	+	++
Planes in any orientation	+	+	–	+	+	++
Study of the entire vessel	–	++	++	–	+	++
Resolution without contrast	+	–	+	++	++	++
Dynamic studies	–	++	–	++	++	++
Flow quantitation	–	++	–	+	+	++
Wall analysis	–	+	++	++	++	++
Comprehensible interpretation	–	+	++	+	++	++
Availability and reasonable cost	++	+	++	++	+	+

this type of sequence is characterized by high signal intensity of the solid structures, while circulating blood, on the other hand, presents a characteristic absence of signal due to the phenomenon of wash-out (time elapsed between the two acquisition excitations in which the spin echo modality is based and which allows the blood flow excited during the first excitation to abandon the study plane before the second acquisition is taken)[2]. This causes a marked, natural contrast between the aorta walls and normal blood flow ("dark blood"), although even under conditions of normal blood velocity, intraluminal flow signals are frequently registered in some slices due to the fact that the blood flow may have been saturated during previous slices (Figure 3.2), a phenomenon which is produced naturally in cases of stasis or abnormally slow circulation.

With the gradient echo technique, an acquisition strategy is applied that provides images of sufficient quality for the morphological study and, furthermore, it offers the possibility of dynamic studies by linking a series of 12 to 30 images of the same slice acquired during different phases of the cardiac cycle (cine MRI)[3]. The technique is also extremely sensitive to blood flow, which has the greatest signal intensity ("bright blood"), this constituting an important complement in the study of aortic disease states (Figure 3.3). Although gradient echo sequences provide less contrast of the static structures than those of spin echo, in the case

of aortic study, they have two advantages: 1) distinguishing between a phenomenon of thrombosis and slow blood flow, a distinction that is occasionally difficult to make with the spin echo technique (Figures 3.4A-B); 2) the direct visualization of blood flow turbulence, which causes the characteristic signal void that contrasts naturally with laminar blood flow[4] (Figure 3.5).

The variants of the gradient echo technique, known as fast gradient echo, in which the acquisition of the lines that compose the image is accomplished in the form of "packets" (segmentation), permit the acquisition of an image in 12 to 16 seconds. This can also be done during an apnea phase of the patient, which significantly reduces the interference of respiratory movements with the image[5] (Figure 3.6). Although the acquisition of these rapid sequences produces a greater number of artifacts than the conventional ones in the aortic study[6], they may be applied simultaneously with the administration of a paramagnetic contrast agent, this greatly improving the definition of of the vessel[7]. On the other hand, with the aid of computerized tridimensional reconstruction techniques applied to tomographies of the aorta obtained with paramagnetic contrast, images can be obtained in which the vessel can be imaged as if viewed from within. As the observer can then move at will along the aortic course, a technique which has come to be known as virtual aortic endoscopy[8].

FIGURE 3.1A

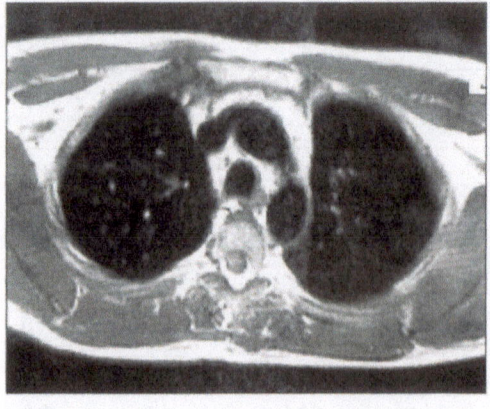

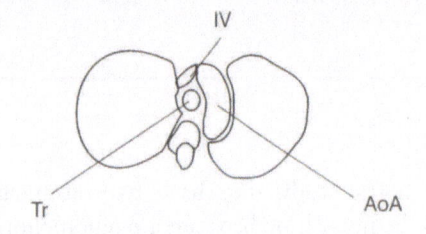

FIGURE 3.1C

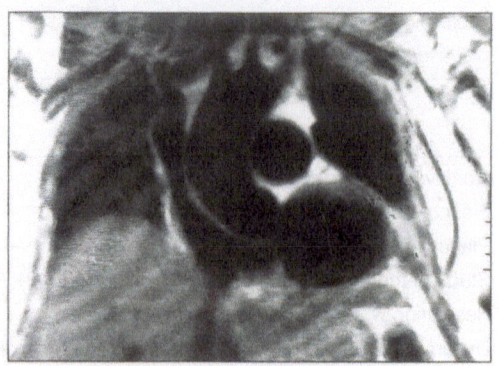

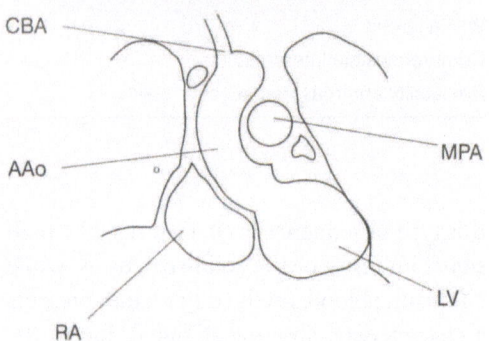

FIGURE 3.1B

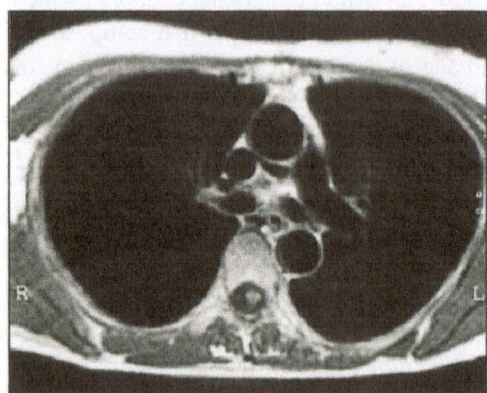

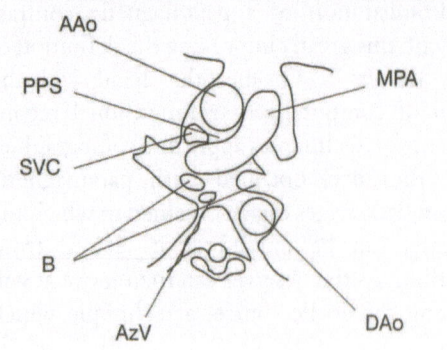

F. 3.1. Normal spin echo planes for the study of the aorta: (A) superior thoracic axial. AoA: aortic arch; IV: innominate vein; Tr: trachea. (B) middle thoracic axial. AAo: ascending aorta; AzV: azygous vein; B: bronchi; DAo: descending aorta; MPA: main pulmonary artery; PPS: posterior pericardial sinus; SVC: superior vena cava. (C) thoracic coronal. AAo: ascending aorta; CBA: common brachiocepahlic artery; LV: left ventricle; MPA: main pulmonary artery; RA: right atrium. (D) thoracic sagittal. AoA: aortic arch; LA: left atrium; LV: left ventricle; RV: right ventricle. E: superior abdominal axial. DAo: descending aorta; SVC: superior vena cava.

F. 3.2. Thoracic axial plane in spin echo in a normal subject. Note the presence of a flow signal in the interior of the descending aorta. AAo: ascending aorta; DAo: descending aorta; B: bronchi; MPA: main pulmonary artery; SVC: superior vena cava.

F. 3.3. Oblique sagittal plane using gradient echo oriented on the plane of the aorta. Ao: aorta; CBA: common brachiocephalic artery; LA: left atrium; PA: pulmonary artery; RA: right atrium.

FIGURE 3.1D

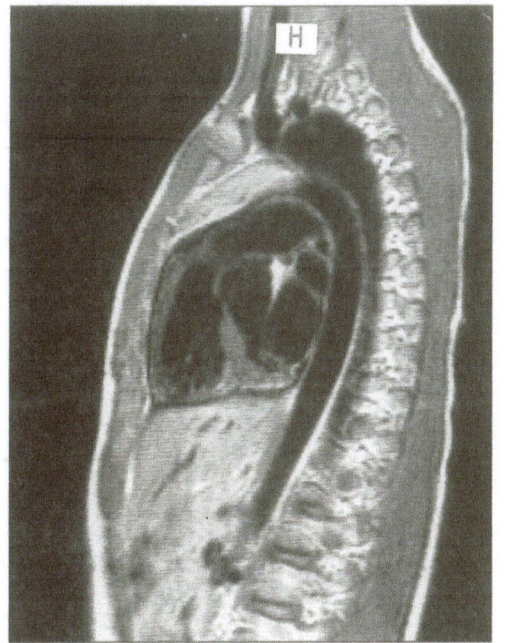

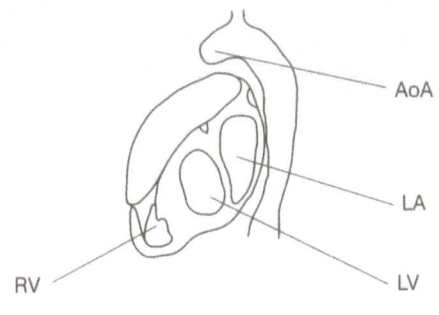

AoA

LA

RV

LV

FIGURE 3.1E

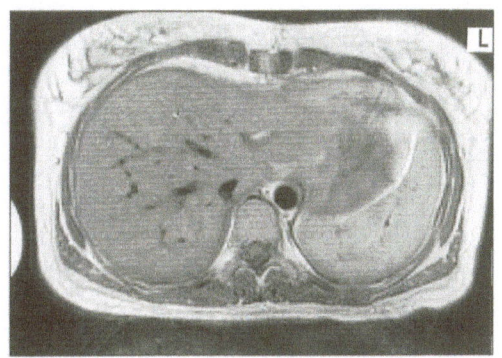

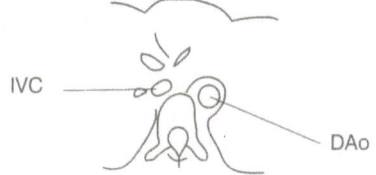

IVC

DAo

FIGURE 3.2

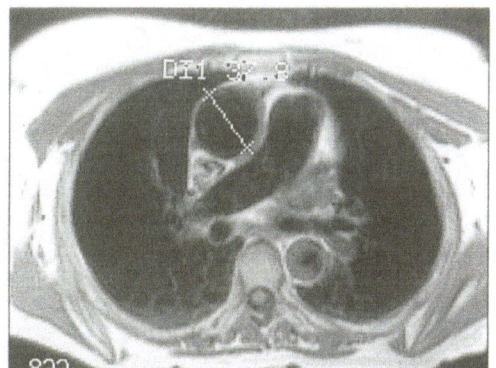

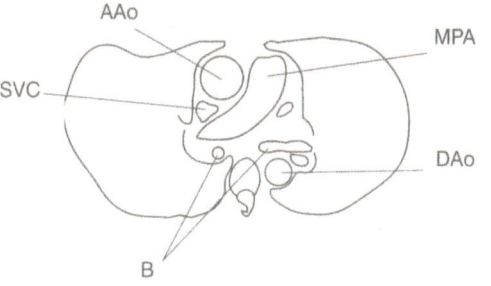

AAo

MPA

SVC

DAo

B

FIGURE 3.3

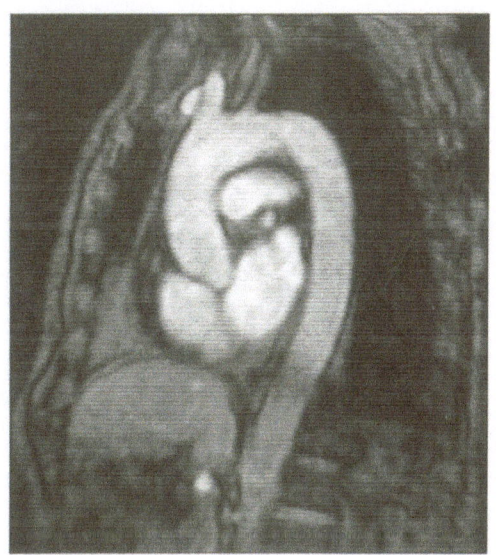

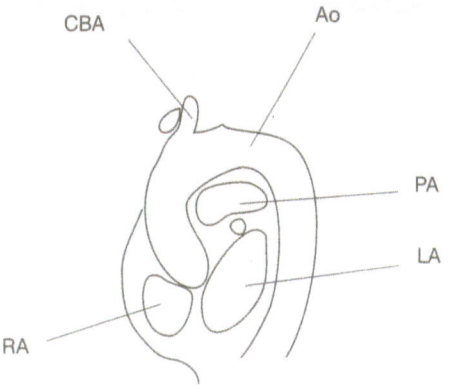

CBA

Ao

PA

LA

RA

FIGURE 3.4A

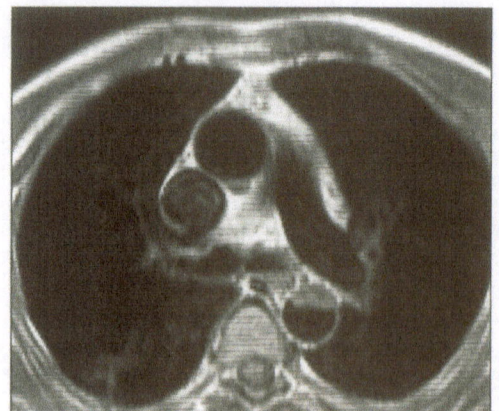

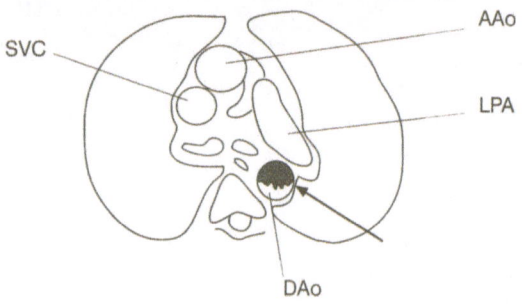

SVC

AAo

LPA

DAo

FIGURE 3.5

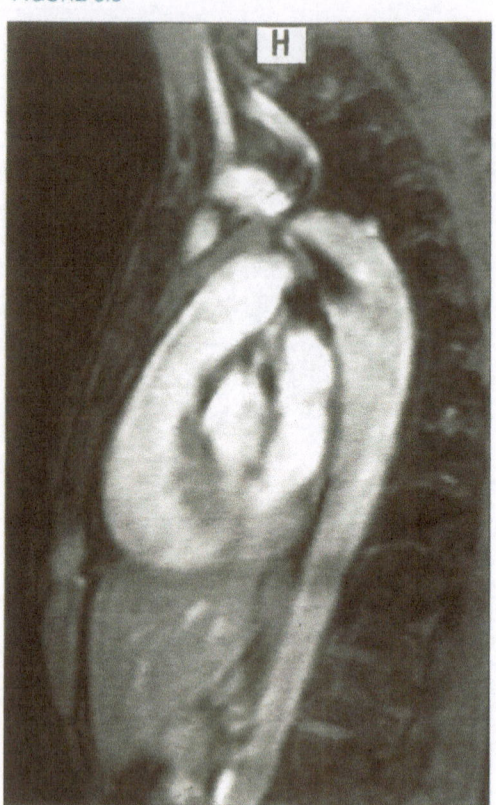

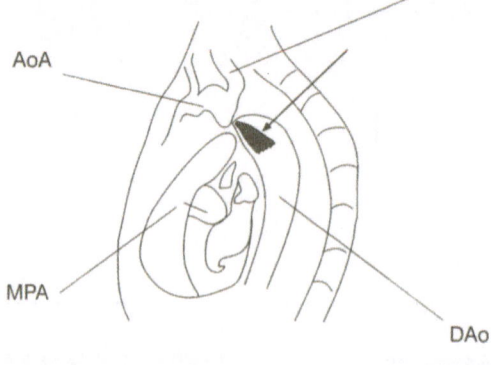

LSA

AoA

MPA

DAo

FIGURE 3.4B

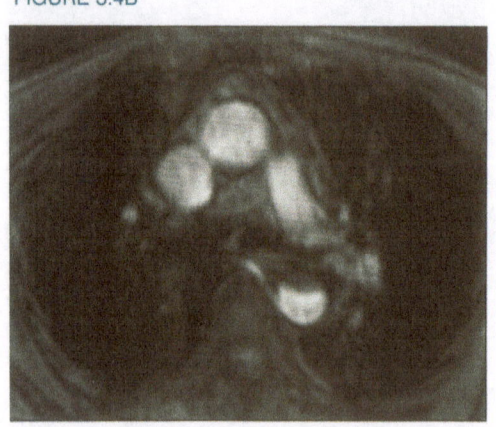

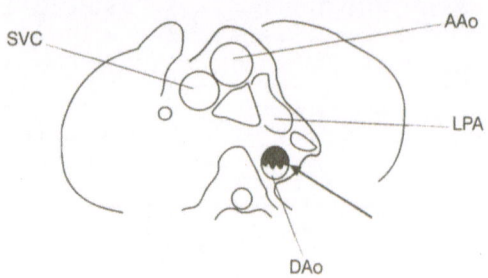

SVC

AAo

LPA

DAo

F. 3.4.   Mural thrombosis (arrrows) in the interior of the descending aorta. (A) axial plane in spin echo. (B) axial plane in gradient echo at the same level. AAo: ascending aorta; DAo: descending aorta; LPA: left pulmonary artery; SVC: superior vena cava.

F. 3.5.   Oblique sagittal plane in gradient echo in a case of coarctation of the aorta in which a phenomenon of signal void can be observed (arrow), indicative of flow turbulence due to the coarctation. DAo: descending aorta; LSA: left subclavian artery; AoA: aortic arch; MPA: main pulmonary artery.

3.2 Aortic Aneurysm

The dilatation of a variable extension of the aorta is a frequent problem, whether it is over the base of a congenital defect of the connective tissue, as in Marfan's syndrome[9], or as part of the spectrum of atherosclerosis[10]. MRI has become the technique of choice for the study of aortic aneurysm due to the advantages it provides, such as those already mentioned. By means of simple spin echo sequences, it is possible, with the correct orientations, to obtain images of the entire extension of the vessel. Eventual dilatations of the caliber (Figures 3.7–3.9) can be identified, as well as the possible presence of intraluminal thrombosis (Figure 3.10).

Of particular interest is the possibility of carrying out follow-up studies with exact and reproducible measurements of the dimensions of the aneurysm, which result in important implications concerning the decision as to whether or not a surgical resection is required, as the decision to consider surgery is based on the diameter of the aortic lumen in the aneurysm.

3.3 Aortic Dissection and Related Entities

a. Strategy for the study of aortic dissection by MRI

A first important aspect to be considered when acute aortic dissection is suspected is the clinical situation of the patient. It must be kept in mind that MRI equipment is generally not located near intensive care units and that the study requires almost one hour for a complete examination. Also, during this time the immediate access to the patient is restricted, both for patient monitoring and for an eventual emergency medical treatment. Therefore, a careful clinical evaluation of each case is imperative before deciding to carry out the MRI examination, which can even be canceled if the patient is judged to be unstable. In this sense, the experience of groups that have carried out MRI studies on a long series of patients with dissection is of interest: in these studies no complications

attributable to isolation have been reported in any case[11], as long as the basic precautions we have mentioned were observed.

The study can be satisfactorily carried out, as has been noted, by conventional means that are available in practically all MRI systems. The recommended sequences are those which are detailed below:

1. Thoracic coronal localizing planes

2. Thoracic axial spin echo series

This series permits the acquisition of transverse images of the thoracic aorta. In the case of dissection, the presence of the dissected intimal layer in the aortic lumen can be detected (Figure 3.11), as well as its extension along the vessel. It is also easy to determine the diameters of the different aortic segments. Although the absence of signal in the interior of the false lumen confidently indicates that circulating flow exists at this level, the presence of a relatively intense signal may correspond to either a condition of slow flow or to the presence of thrombosis of the false lumen (Figure 3.12 and 3.13).

3. Thoracic coronal spin echo series

This series, useful as a complement to the previous one, provides longitudinal images of the ascending and descending aorta, as well as transverse images of the aortic arch, which facilitate the localization of the dissection site (Figure 3.14).

4. Cine MRI sequence in gradient echo on the aortic plane

This sequence can be programmed along one of the axial planes where both the ascending and descending aorta are visualized (Figure 3.12) by orienting the slice plane over the ascending and descending aorta. The information this sequence provides is of special interest because the presentation of the images is the same as that offered by conventional contrast aortography, a view which both clinicians and surgeons are familiar with. In case of dissection, this sequence is an important complement to the spin echo series as, in addition to visualizing the presence and extension of the intimal membrane, it also helps in the identification of flow conditions of the false lumen (Figure 3.15).

FIGURE 3.6

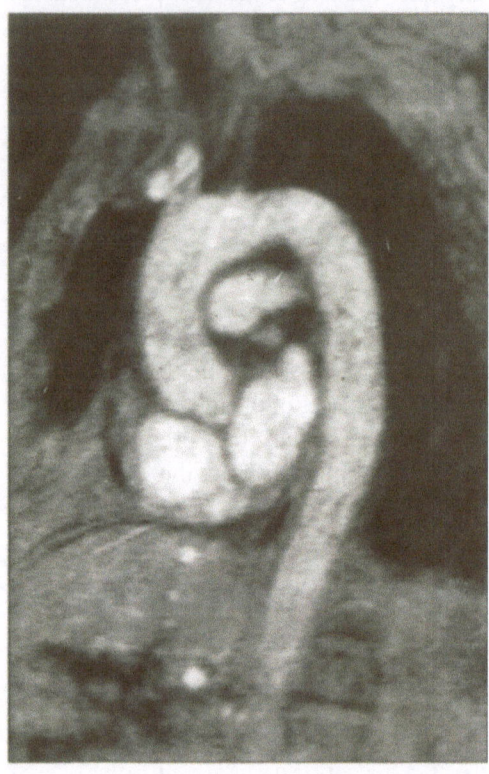

FIGURE 3.7

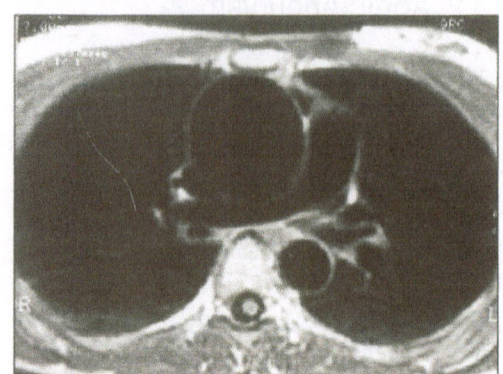

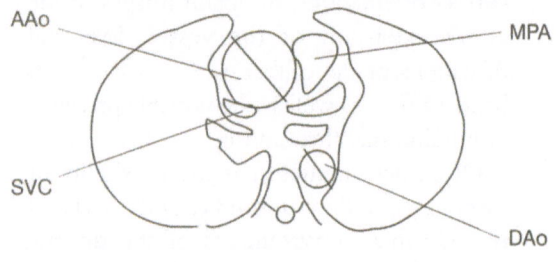

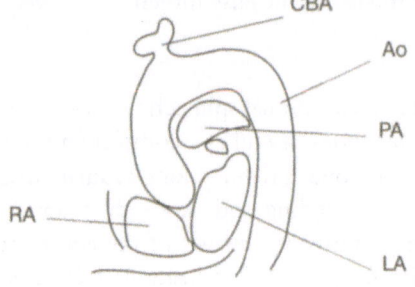

FIGURE 3.8

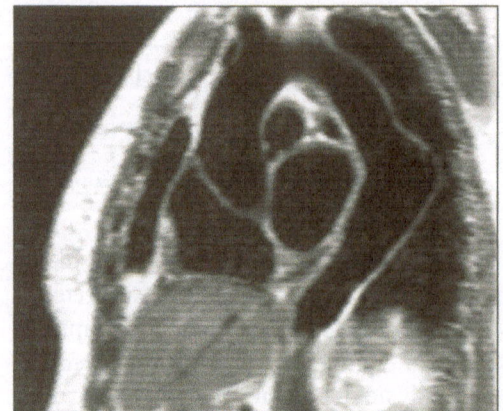

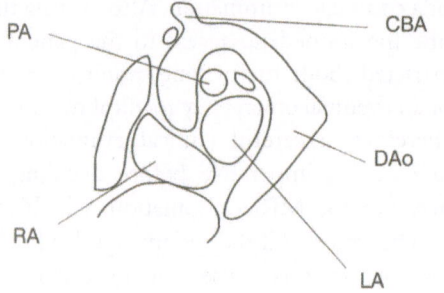

F. 3.6.   Oblique sagittal plane using a fast technique of segmented k-space oriented on the aortic plane corresponding to the same plane depicted in Figure 3.3. Ao: aorta; CBA: common brachiocephalic artery; LA: left atrium; PA: pulmonary artery; RA: right atrium.

F. 3.7.   Axial plane in spin echo in a case of annulo-aortic ectasia. AAo: ascending aorta; DAo: descending aorta; MPA: main pulmonary artery; SVC: superior vena cava.

F. 3.8.   Oblique sagittal plane in spin echo on the aortic plane in a case of fusiform aneurysm of the descending aorta. CBA: common brachiocephalic artery; DAo: descending aorta; LA: left atrium; PA: pulmonary artery; RA: right atrium.

FIGURE 3.9

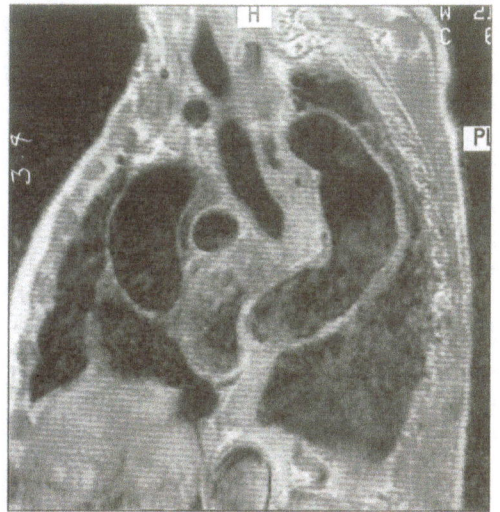

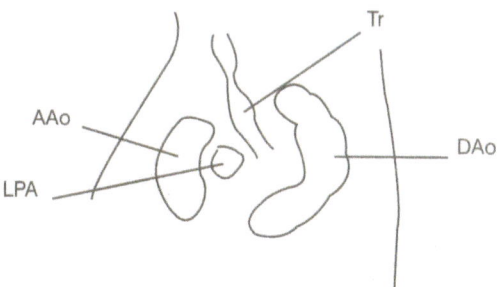

FIGURE 3.10A

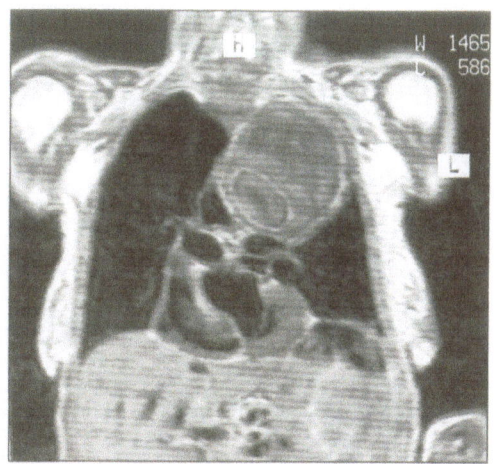

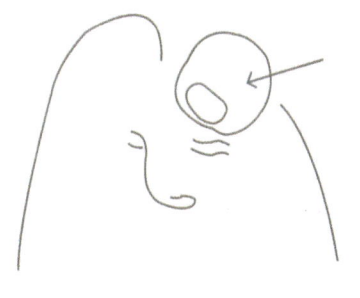

FIGURE 3.10B

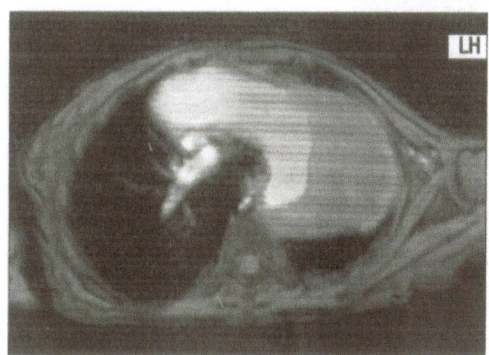

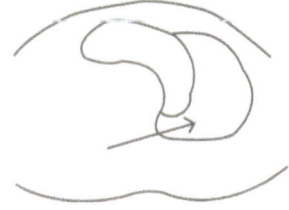

F. 3.9. Oblique sagittal plane in spin echo in a case of atherosclerotic aneurysm of the thoracic aorta with dilatation and tortuous vessel course. AAo: ascending aorta; DAo: descending aorta; LPA: left pulmonary artery; Tr: trachea.

F. 3.10 (A) Thoracic coronal plane in spin echo in a case of atherosclerotic aneurysm of the aortic arch with mural thrombosis in its interior (arrow). (B) Axial gradient-echo in the same patient showing that the aneurysm involves the distal half of the arch, the difference between flowing blood (bright signal) and thrombosis (dark signal) of the aneurysmal sac (arrow) being evident.

FIGURE 3.11

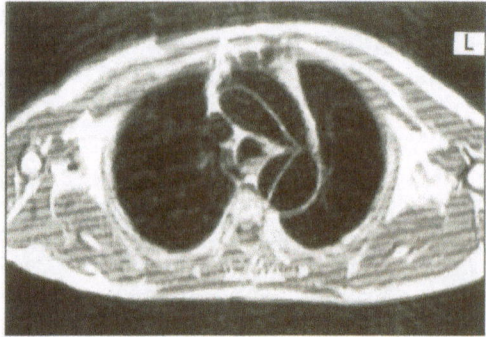

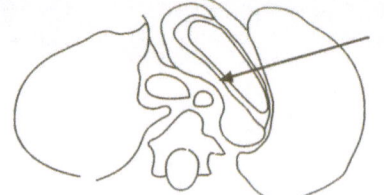

FIGURE 3.13

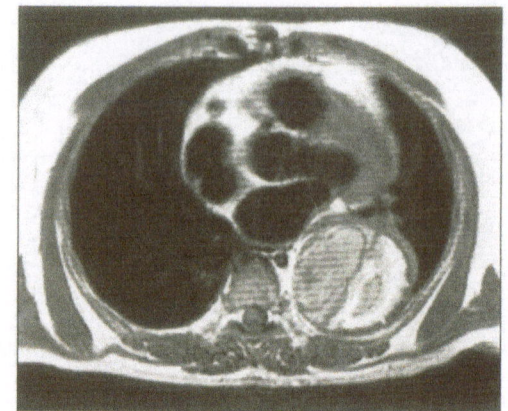

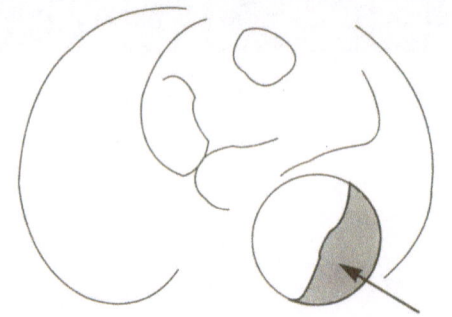

FIGURE 3.12

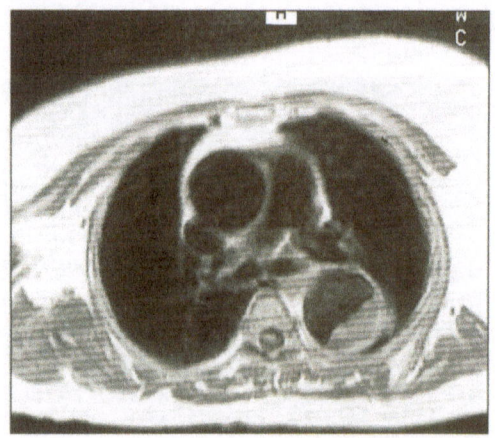

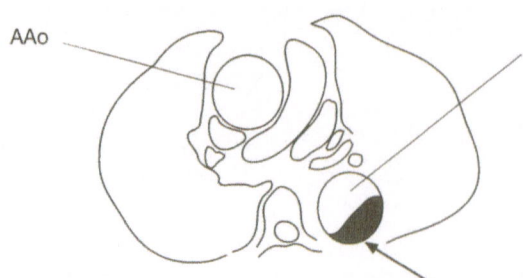

AAo

DAo

FIGURE 3.14

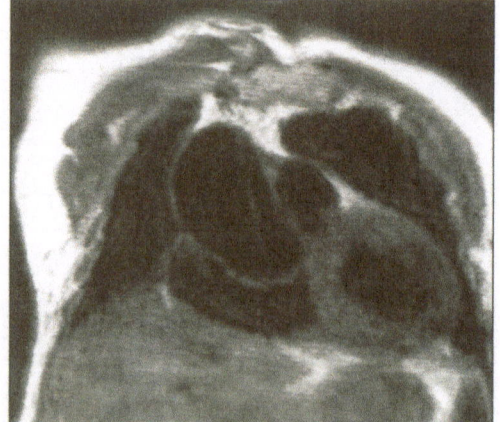

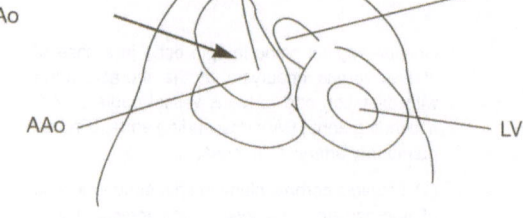

MPA

AAo

LV

5. Cine gradient echo along a longitudinal axis of the left ventricle

With this series a left ventriculography is obtained that provides important information in the case of a type A aortic dissection: it allows the estimation of left ventricular function and also helps in ruling out the presence of a pericardial effusion or of an eventual aortic regurgitation (Figure 3.16).

6. Axial abdominal spin echo sequence

This series, by allowing the study of the possible implication of the visceral arterial trunks, is important in case the dissection has extended itself to the abdominal aorta (Figure 3.17). It must be kept in mind that the implementation of this series may cause the patient to be repositioned in the equipment tube in order to obtain new localizing planes, which entails a consequent time delay.

Although a complete study, including all the previously mentioned sequences, may easily take an hour, the decision to limit the study, depending on the information obtained in each sequence and the type of dissection, is left to the judgement of the operator. Thus, a type A dissection limited to the ascending aorta would probably not require an abdominal study, while a dynamic study of the left ventricle would not be necessary in a type B dissection.

b. Differential diagnosis of aortic dissection by MRI

Since the cornerstone of the diagnosis of aortic dissection is the detection of the dissected intimal–medial membrane, it is important to be aware of some of the possible sources of uncertainty concerning its recognition using MRI. On one hand, there are normal anatomical structures or even artifacts that can lead to a false-positive diagnosis[12]. On the other hand, atypical forms of a true dissection, although they manifest themselves clinically as such, may not be recognized and lead to a false-negative diagnosis[13].

The images which can most frequently lead to a false-positive diagnosis of dissection using MRI are, in the first place, those which depict the left venous brachiocephalic trunk (Figure 3.1A), which runs in close relation to the anterior aspect of the aortic arch and which is, of course, normal, or those which depict the presence of the posterior aortic pericardium reflection (Figure 3.1B). In other cases the problem comes from the presence of intraluminal flow signals, already mentioned, or artifacts produced by the presence of periaortic fat, which is frequent in those systems with greater field strength (Figure 3.18). In general, all these potential causes of confusion create few difficulties, since the possibility of comparing slices at different levels permits its easy recognition by a clinician with a certain degree of experience.

It is of greater importance to be able to recognize the possible atypical presentations of dissection, those in which a false-negative diagnosis may be made using MRI when a dissected membrane cannot be identified. Thus, although the detection of such a membrane in the interior of an aortic lumen with an otherwise normal caliber or showing no great dilatation is what is most frequently found, a proportion of patients present with the so-called dissection "without rupture"[14] or aortic intramural hematoma. It occurs in up to 13% of the cases of dissection, a percentage which has been demonstrated in clinical[15] as well as in autopsy studies[16]. In these cases, a thickening of the aortic wall of crescent shape or circumferential form has been observed which does not generally deform the circular morphology of the aortic lumen. It displays a signal of intermediate intensity which corresponds to the parietal

---

F. 3.11.   Axial plane in spin echo showing aortic dissection (arrow) in the arch.

F. 3.12.   Axial plane in spin echo in a case of dissection of the descending aorta with a high intensity signal in the interior of the false lumen (arrow). AAo: ascending aorta; DAo: descending aorta.

F. 3.13.   Axial plane in spin echo showing dissection in an enlarged descending aorta where high signal intensity is present at both lumens: the one with the highest intensity (arrow) corresponds to a probably thrombosed false lumen while the true lumen exhibits a slightly less intense signal due to low flow.

F. 3.13.   Coronal plane in spin echo showing dissection in the ascending aorta where rupture of the intimal membrane is detected (arrow). AAo: ascending aorta; MPA: main pulmonary artery; LV: left ventricle.

FIGURE 3.15

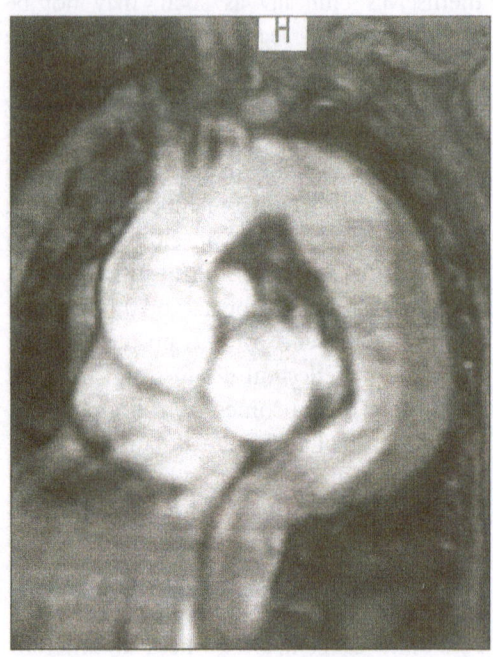

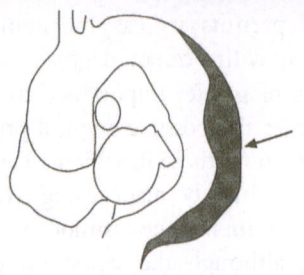

FIGURE 3.16

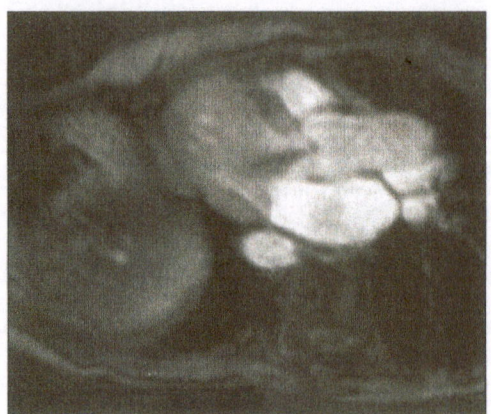

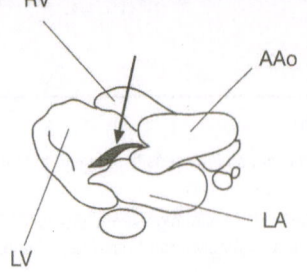

RV

AAo

LV

LA

FIGURE 3.17A

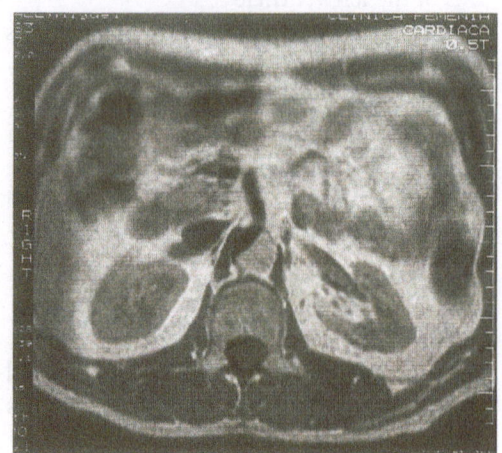

SMA

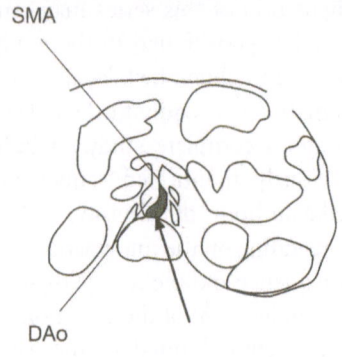

DAo

FIGURE 3.17B

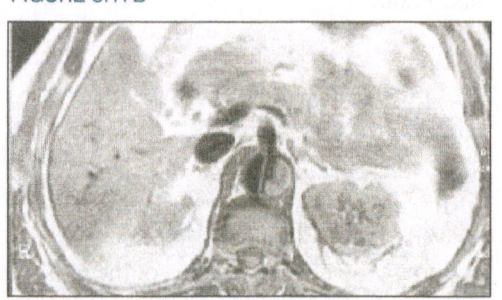

SMA

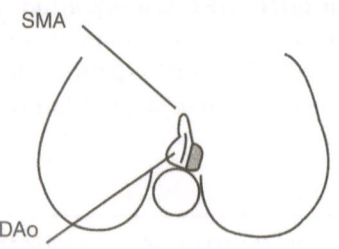

DAo

hematoma (Figure 3.19). This type of image must be distinguished from other pathological forms, specifically from a true dissection with thrombosis of the false lumen, which usually displays deformation of the aortic lumen (Figure 3.12). The distinction must be made as well from an atherosclerotic aneurysm with mural thrombosis in its interior, in which an important dilatation of the aorta is present (Figure 3.10). In these cases the information provided by other imaging techniques may be useful, such as an echocardiography or a CT, fundamentally to detect the presence of calcium in the internal wall of the membrane, which identifies that membrane as the true intima of the aortic wall.

Recognition of the aortic intramural hematoma is of great importance, since it has the same clinical implications as dissection and, in fact, 30% of cases of hematoma can develop into dissection[17]. It has been postulated that the initial phenomenon of dissection may be a hemorrhage of the *vasa vasorum* in the media of the vessel and not a rupture of the intima membrane, the eventual intimal rupture occurring in fact after the intramural hemorrage (Figure 3.20). The existence of intramural hematoma has long been known, although it is frequently not detected by contrast aortography due to the absence of two permeable lumens in the aorta, its importance having been highlighted after the introduction of CT and MRI. Furthermore, since it constitutes a true clinical variant of dissection, the relevant issue seems to be the detection of the presence of an acute aortic disease, whether it is a dissection or a hematoma, and to take clinical measures without waiting to contrast the anatomy of the process with an angio-hemodynamic study[18].

A particular form of acute aortic disease is the so-called aortic parietal ulcer[19], which has a pathogenetic mechanism different from dissection or intramural hematoma. In this case it is not a process of degeneration of the media of the artery, but rather a continuous erosion of an atherosclerotic plaque that penetrates beyond the limits of the internal elastic membrane[20], which may form a localized hematoma and progress toward the formation of a pseudoaneurysm or even an aortic parietal rupture. Its atherosclerotic origin conditions its presentation in elderly patients, normally in the descending aorta[21]. Given the relatively infrequent character of the aortic penetrating ulcer, its variable presentation form, often clinically silent and its morphological versatility, the prognosis has not been established and at this time the most appropriate diagnostic technique cannot be advanced[22]. It is to be hoped, nevertheless, that MRI will be useful also in this sense[23] (Figure 3.21).

These different morphological forms of acute aortic disease may be eventually present in the same patient. It is in these cases where the usefulness of MRI is most evident (Figures 3.22), taking advantage of the integral study of the entire aorta it permits.

References

1. Abernethy LJ, Szezepura AK, Fletcher J, Fitzpatrick JD, Stevens A. Cost effectiveness of magnetic resonance imaging. Br Med J 1992; 304: 183.

2. von Schulthess GK, Fisher M, Crooks LE, Higgins CB. Gated MR imaging of the heart: intracardiac signals in patients and healthy subjects. Radiology 1985; 156: 125–32.

F. 3.15. Oblique sagittal plane in gradient echo over the aortic plane. It corresponds to the same case as that in Figure 3.12; the presence of thrombosis at the level of the false lumen (arrow) is confirmed by the persistence in this sequence of the high signal intensity already observed in the spin echo image.

F. 3.16. Study using gradient echo oriented on a longitudinal plane of the left ventricle (presented here as is usually displayed in the parasternal longitudinal echocardiographic view); a phenomenon of signal void corresponding to aortic valvular insufficiency is detected (arrow). LA: left atrium; AAo: ascending aorta; RV: right ventricle; LV: left ventricle.

F. 3.17. (A) Axial abdominal plane in spin echo in a case of aortic dissection. The false lumen of the dissection can be identified by the increase in signal intensity in this area; it may also be observed how the superior mesenteric artery originates from the true lumen (arrow). (B) The same plane in a different patient where the mesenteric artery is seen to be compromised by the dissection. DAo: descending aorta; SMA: superior mesenteric artery.

FIGURE 3.18

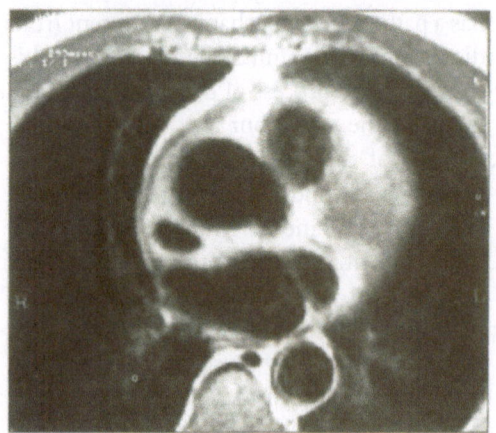

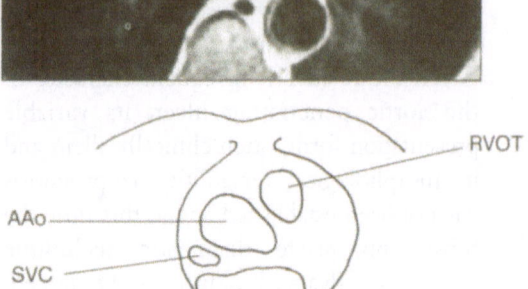

RVOT

AAo

SVC

LA

DAo

FIGURE 3.20A

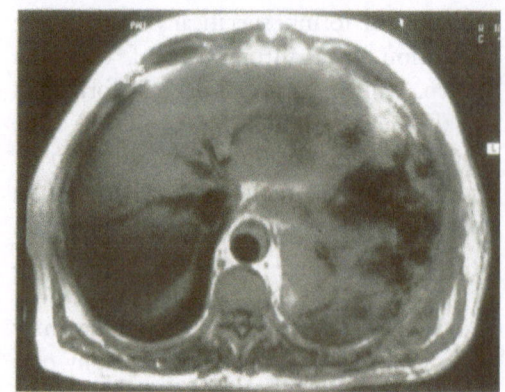

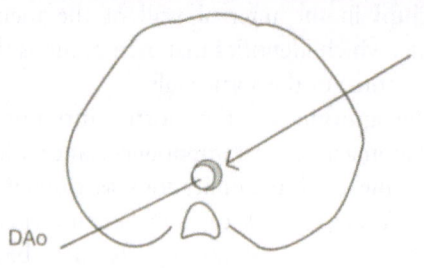

DAo

FIGURE 3.19

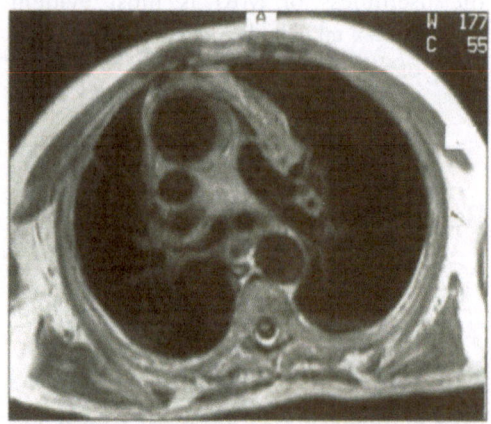

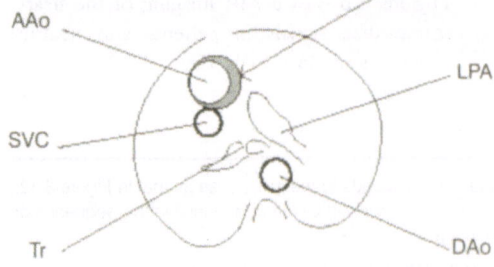

AAo

SVC

Tr

LPA

DAo

FIGURE 3.20B

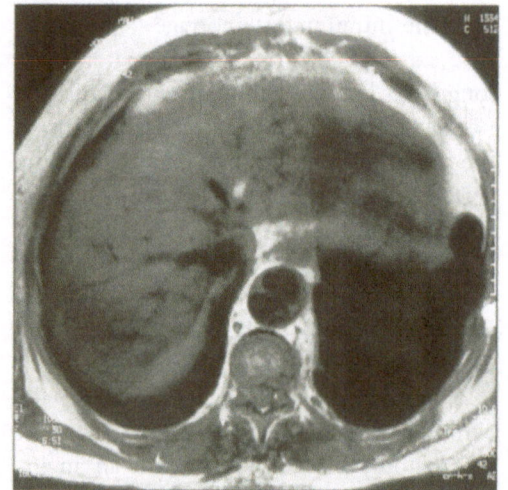

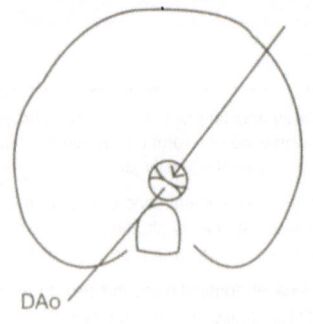

DAo

FIGURE 3.21A

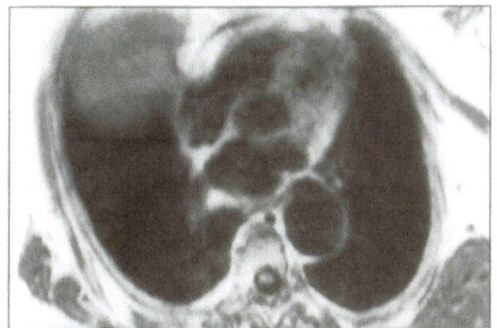

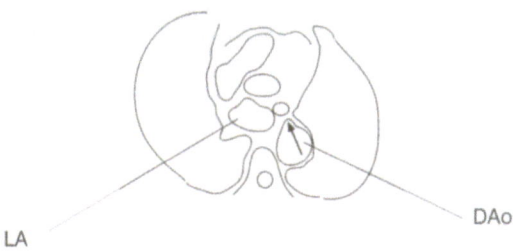

LA

DAo

FIGURE 3.21B

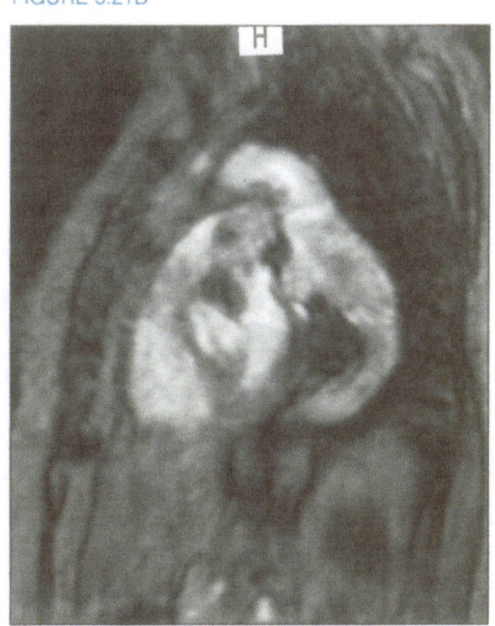

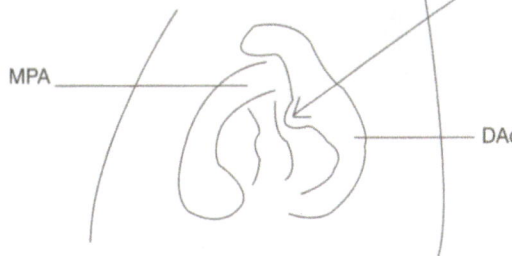

MPA

DAo

F. 3.18. Thoracic axial plane in spin echo: an artifact can be observed in the interior of the descending aorta (arrow) due to the presence of periaortic fat. AAo: ascending aorta; DAo: descending aorta; LA: left atrium; RV: right ventricle; SVC: superior vena cava.

F. 3.19. Axial spin echo image showing a crescent shaped thickening of the ascending aortic wall exhibiting high signal intensity (arrow) in a case of intramural hematoma. AAo: ascending aorta; DAo: descending aorta; LPA: left pulmonary artery; SVC: superior vena cava; Tr: trachea.

F. 3.20. (A) Intramural hematoma (arrow) of the descending aorta in a spin echo image. (B) A comparable study in the same plane patient one year later, showing the presence of a true dissection (arrow) with evidence of flow patency at both lumens. DAo: descending aorta

F. 3.21. (A) Axial plane in spin echo showing a penetrating ulcer in the descending aorta (arrow). (B) Sagittal gradient-echo in the same patient, showing the longitudinal extension of the ulcer (arrow). DAo: descending aorta LA: left atrium; MPA: main pulmonary artery.

FIGURE 3.22A

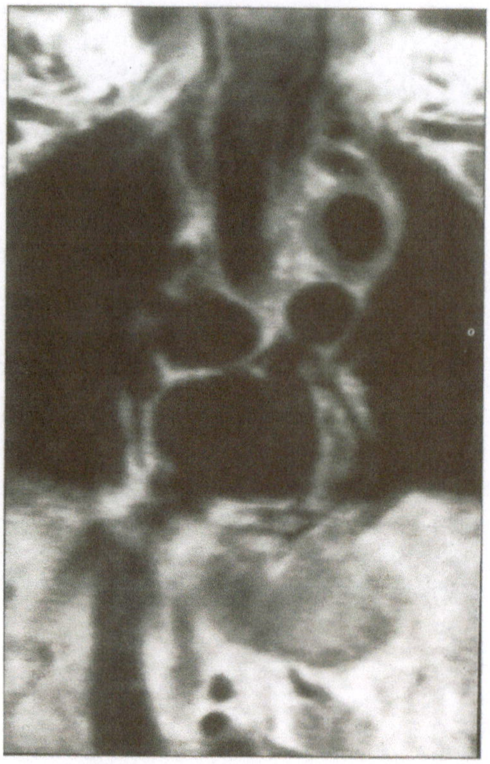

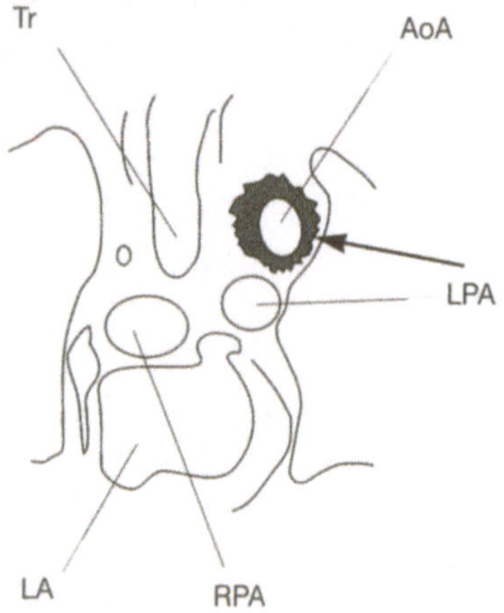

FIGURE 3.22A

FIGURE 3.22B

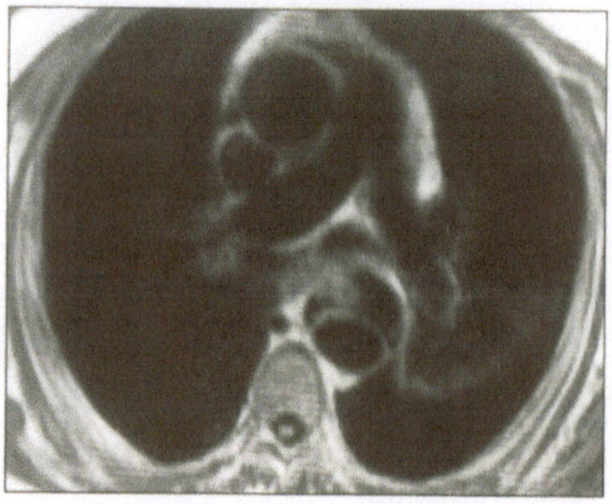

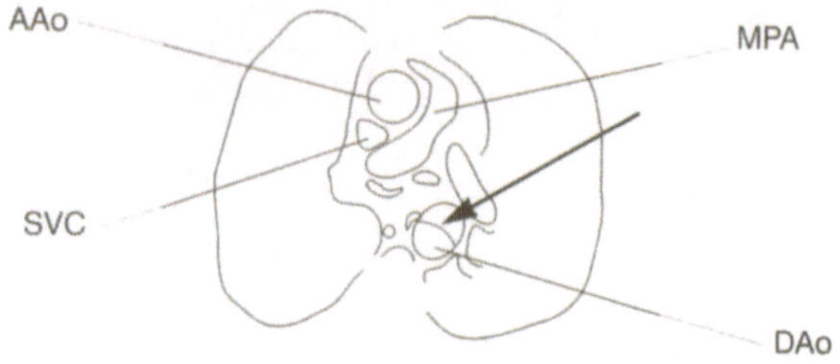

FIGURE 3.22C

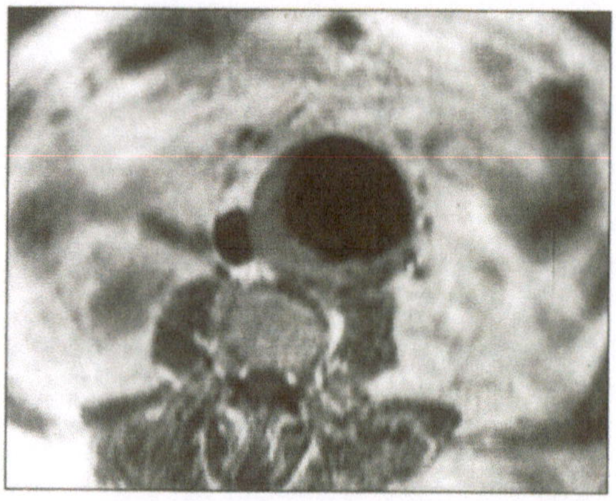

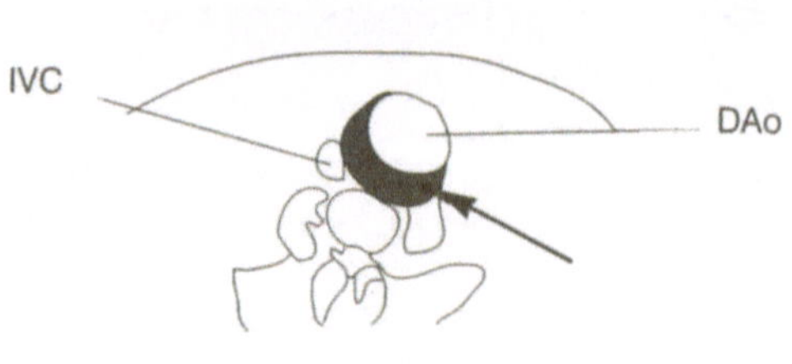

F. 3.22. Spin echo images at different levels from the same patient. (A) Coronal plane showing an increase in the thickness of the wall of the aortic arch due to intramural hematoma (arrow); (B) Axial thoracic plane in which a dissection of the descending aorta is observed (arrow) with patency at both lumens; (C) Abdominal axial plane showing an arteriosclerotic aneurysm with mural thrombosis (arrow). AoA: aortic arch; DAo: descending aorta; IVC: inferior vena cava; LA: left atrium; LPA: left pulmonary artery; MPA: main pulmonary artery; RPA: right pulmonary artery; SVC: superior vena cava; Tr: trachea.

3. Sechtem U, Pflugfelder PW, White RD, et al. Cine MR imaging: potential for the evaluation of cardiovascular function. Am J Röentgenol 1987; 148: 239–46.

4. Pettigrew RI. Cardiovascular imaging techniques. In: Stark DD, Bradley WB, ed. Magnetic resonance imaging. St Louis: Mosby-Year Book; 1992: 1605–51.

5. Atkinson DJ, Edelman RR. Cineangiography of the heart in a single breath hold with a segmented Turbo FLASH sequence. Radiology 1991; 178: 357–60.

6. Hartnell GG, Finn JP, Zenni M, et al. MR imaging of the thoracic aorta: comparison of spin-echo, angiographic, and breath-hold techniques. Radiology 1994; 191: 697–704.

7. Revel D, Loubeyre P, Delignette A, Douek P, Amiel M. Contrast-enhanced magnetic resonance tomoangiography: a new imaging technique for studying thoracic great vessels. Magn Reson Imaging 1993; 11: 1101–5.

8. Davis CP, Ladd ME, Romanowski BJ, Wildermuth S, Knoplioch JF, Debatin JF. Human aorta: preliminary results with virtual endoscopy based on three-dimensional MR imaging data sets. Radiology 1996; 199: 37–40.

9. Pyeritz RE. Marfan syndrome. N Engl J Med 1990; 323: 987–9.

10. Reed D, Reed C, Stemmermann G, Hayashi T. Are aortic aneurysms caused by atherosclerosis? Circulation 1992 ; 85: 205–11.

11. Nienaber CA, von Kodolitsch Y, Nicolas V, et al. The diagnosis of thoracic aortic dissection by noninvasive imaging procedures. N Engl J Med 1993; 328: 1–9.

12. Solomon SL, Brown JL, Glazer HS, Mirowitz SA, Lee JKT. Thoracic aortic dissection: pitfalls and artifacts in MR imaging. Radiology 1990; 177: 223–8.

13. Wolff KA, Herold CJ, Tempany CM, Parravano JG, Zerhouni EA. Aortic dissection: atypical patterns seen at MR imaging. Radiology 1991; 181: 489–95.

14. Yamada T, Tada S, Harada J. Aortic dissection without intimal rupture: diagnosis with MR imaging and CT. Radiology 1988; 168: 347–52.

15. Nienaber CA, von Kodolitsch Y, Petersen B, et al. Intramural hemorrhage of the thoracic aorta. Diagnostic and therapeutic implications. Circulation 1995; 92: 1465–72.

16. Wilson SK, Hutchins GM. Aortic dissecting aneurysms: causative factors in 204 subjects. Arch Pathol Lab Med 1982; 106: 175–80.

17. Evangelista A, Salas A, Armada E, González-Alujas MT, GarcRa del Castillo H, Soler-Soler J. Does the form of presentation predict the evolution of an aortic haematoma? Eur Heart J 1996; 17 (Abstr. Suppl.): 439.

18. O'Gara PT, DeSanctis RW. Acute aortic dissection and its variants. Toward a common diagnostic and therapeutic approach. Circulation 1995; 92: 1376–8.

19. Kazerooni EA, Bree RL, Williams DM. Penetrating atherosclerotic ulcers of the descending thoracic aorta: evaluation with CT and distinction from aortic dissection. Radiology 1992; 183: 759–65.

20. Stanson AW, Kazmier FJ, Hollier LH, et al. Penetrating atherosclerotic ulcers of the thoracic aorta: natural history and clincopathologic correlations. Ann Vasc Surg 1986; 1: 15–23.

21. Vilacosta I, San Roman JA, Aragoncillo P, et al. Penetrating atherosclerotic aortic ulcer: documentation by transesophageal echocardiography. J Am Coll Cardiol 1998; 32: 83–9.

22. Cooke JP, Kazmier FJ, Orszulak TA. The penetrating aortic ulcer pathologic manifestations, diagnosis and management. Mayo Clin Proc 1988; 63: 718–25.

23. Yucel EK, Steinberg FL, Egglin TK, Geller SC, Waltman AC, Athanasoulis CA. Penetrating aortic ulcers: diagnosis with MR imaging. Radiology 1990; 177: 779–81.

Study of valvular heart disease

4

L.J. JIMÉNEZ-BORREGUERO

4.1 Introduction

Magnetic resonance has proven to be of considerable usefulness in the study of valvular heart disease and in the evaluation of its severity and the associated complications. Although echocardiography continues to be the method of choice in this disease, MRI represents an alternative when echocardiographic results are inconclusive or limited.

The severity of valvular disease can be evaluated by MRI by means of various methods which analyze the behavior of blood flow and the consequences of altered valvular function. Most of the MRI systems are equipped with spin echo ECG-gated sequences and also with cine gradient echo, which are used to perform most of cardiac examinations. The cine gradient echo sequences generate images that permit the phenomena of high flow velocity and turbulence which characterize stenosis and allow valvular regurgitation to be highlighted. Cine loop display of images obtained during different phases of the cardiac cycle provide a dynamic representation of flow behavior in systole and diastole. Laminar flow, within physiological ranges, causes an intense bright signal which highly contrasts with solid structures in the images. High velocity or turbulent flow produced by stenosis or regurgitation manifests itself as signal void and appears as black or dark grey areas within the normal flow. The intensity and extension of the signal of blood turbulence depends on the technical parameters selected, among which echo time (TE) and spatial resolution stand out. Thus, long TE are sensitive to low turbulences and to low velocity ranges, and are, therefore, useful for the study of venous flow. Short TE are sensitive to high degrees of turbulence and to high velocity ranges and are used for the analysis of significant valvular stenosis or regurgitation.

4.2 Velocity Calculation and Flow Quantitation

With velocity-encoded cine MRI, quantitative velocity maps can be obtained in three spatial directions and with the desired orientation without window restrictions and with a wide range of flow velocity values. The MRI sequences most widely used for this purpose are known as phase contrast images (Figure 4.1), and are based on the principle that the movement of any structure containing hydrogen generates a phase shift of the radiofrequency waves in the presence of a specific sequence of magnetic gradients and stimuli. The dephasing of the radio-frequency waves is directly proportional to the velocity of the structure or fluid under study. The obtained maps represent in dark grey the velocity directed in one direction (e.g. caudo-cranial) and in white or bright tones the movement in the opposite direction (e.g. cranio-caudal). As is the case with the other sequences, the cine velocity maps are also obtained from a specific number of cardiac cycles.

In valvular stenosis the flow velocity can be analyzed by two methods. The simplest one consists of applying cine MRI velocity mapping in multiple contiguous slices parallel to the valvular plane in the receiving cardiac chamber. The velocity is encoded in a direction perpendicular to the study plane in such a way that in some of the selected slices the peak velocity value will be obtained. This occurs in the *vena contracta* region, that is observed at a distance of a few millimeters over the plane of the stenosis, where the lines of flow velocity present their point of peak concentration.

The maximal velocity is also registered in the slice planes that coincide with both the flow direction and the velocity encoding in one or two spatial directions. In order to avoid underestimation of the recorded velocity, it is recommended that the encoded velocity direction coincide with that of the stenotic jet. Previous representation of flow turbulence with cine gradient echo images provides a reference for an accurate alignment of the cine velocity maps.

Velocity encoded through the imaging plane, on an axial slice of great arteries or veins, is needed for the calculation of flow. The average velocity of the flow in the lumen of the vessel, multiplied by the area of its section, gives a precise calculation of the instantaneous flow[1]. The flow value obtained in each phase of the cardiac cycle is registered on a graph of flow plotted against time (Figure 4.2) the area under the curve representing the flow volume. Besides the quantitative estimation of velocity and flow values, the presentation in cine format of the images provides dynamic information on flow.

4.3 Anatomical Evaluation

The appropriate clinical management of valvular heart disease requires information not only on the clinical situation of the patient and the severity of the valve lesion but also on its consequences on the size and contractile function of the ventricles. MRI provides this information, the cardiac structures being visualized in motion with cine gradient echo that permits the analysis of size, thickness and contractile ventricular function. Spin echo multislice sequences are not as useful in this case due to their static nature, depicting different anatomical levels, each during a different moment of the cardiac cycle.

Direct anatomical valvular imaging by MRI has certain limitations. The valvular leaflets can be examined in motion using cine sequences with gradient echo and the degree of valve thickening can be determined. Although highly fibrous areas appear in black or dark grey as a consequence of the low signal intensity produced by the fibrous tissue, MRI does not differentiate the presence of calcium from fibrosis due to the fact that both generate a similar signal void effect. The valvular leaflets are seen with spin echo or gradient echo techniques (Figure 4.3), but its mobility cannot be studied as appropriately as with echocardiography. Also, the signal void due to the eventual presence of calcium adhering to the valve may be indistinguishable from signals due to moving blood.

MRI has been used however to demonstrate endocardiac vegetations and their complications, such as pseudoaneurysms or abscesses[2,3]. Endocardial vegetations are identified in cine gradient echo as low signal areas in the valvular leaflet moving during systole and diastole. They are differentiated from the flow turbulence secondary to stenosis or valvular insufficiency in that they

FIGURE 4.1 A and B

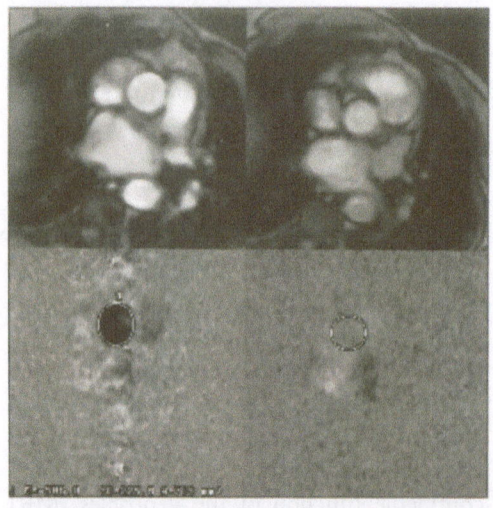

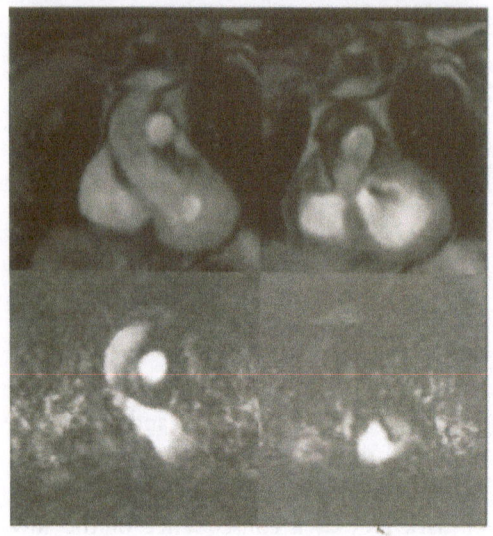

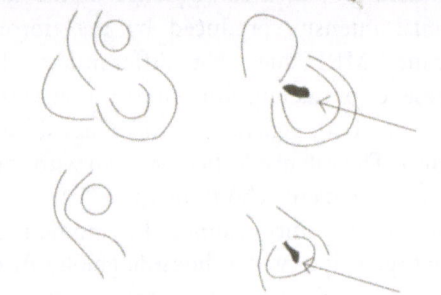

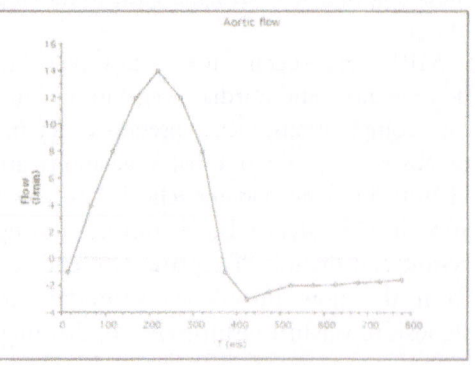

FIGURE 4.2

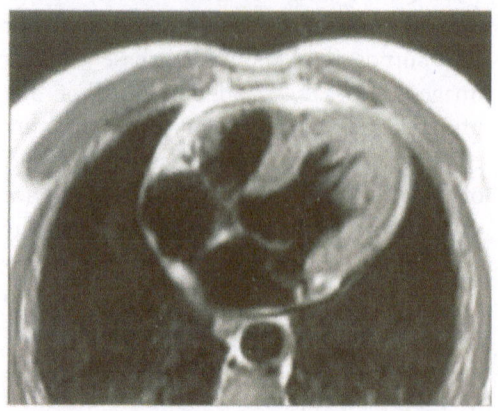

FIGURE 4.3 A and B

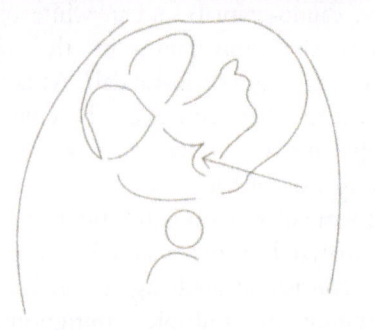

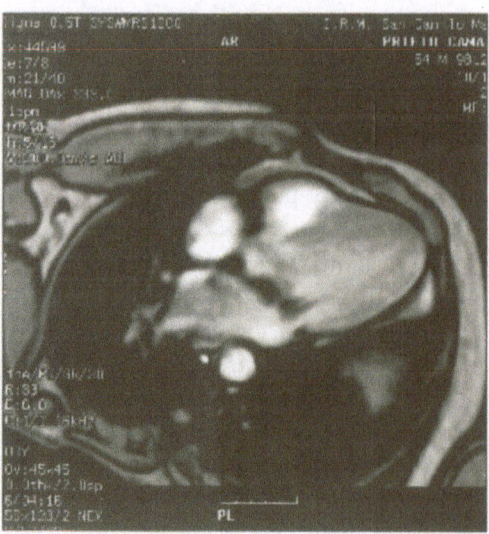

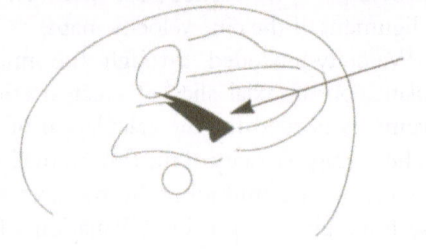

only appear in systole or diastole, respectively, whereas the movement of the vegetations persists during the entire cardiac cycle. In those rare cases in which echocardiography is inconclusive MRI may be an alternative for the diagnosis and evaluation of valvular endocarditis and its complications.

4.4 Aortic Regurgitation

a. Quantitation with cine MRI velocity mapping

Calculation of the regurgitant volume or fraction permits precise quantitation of the severity of valvular aortic insufficiency[4]. The simplest MRI method uses cine velocity maps on a plane axial to the ascending aorta, where at least 16 phases of the cardiac cycle are obtained in order to evaluate flow behavior during ventricular contraction and relaxation. The velocity is encoded through a plane so that the flow velocity over the entire surface of the aortic section can be analyzed. Unlike Doppler echocardiography, which samples blood velocity in a small volume or over a specific line, MRI simultaneously analyzes flow over the entire cross-section of the aorta. This method permits a precise calculation of the flow volume in each phase of the cardiac cycle, which is obtained by multiplying the average velocity of this surface by the area of the section. The values that are obtained are transferred to a flow/time curve that includes both a systole and diastole (Figure 4.2). The planimetry of the area under the diastolic curve of retrograde flow represents the aortic regurgitation volume. The regurgitant fraction is obtained by dividing retrograde

diastolic flow volume by the antegrade systolic one.

In the phase contrast image, the normal flow in the ascending aorta is presented in intense white or black tones (depending on the encoding map), while the absence of an organized retrograde flow in diastole causes a lack of a definite flow signal. Aortic valvular insufficiency produces retrograde aortic flow that is recorded in a tone opposite to that of the anterograde flow in the ascending aorta (Figure 4.4). In MRI systems equipped with cine image sequencing in phase contrast but without velocity quantitation, this finding may be useful to estimate the severity of regurgitation qualitatively.

b. Quantitation of regurgitant volume using Simpson's method

Ventricular volumes can be calculated by series of slices covering the whole body of the ventricular chambers[5]. The sum of the endocardial areas multiplied by the slice thickness permits the volume of the ventricular chamber to be obtained. In order to calculate the end-diastolic volume, all the measurements must be determined in this phase of the cardiac cycle, and the same criterion is used for the systolic volume. The stroke volume (SV) is then obtained as the difference between the end-diastolic and end-systolic volumes. This method can be applied with any MRI system with gradient echo sequences or biphasic spin echo. The rapid sequences that are incorporated into some systems permit a reduction in the examination time. Once both right and left ventricular volumes have been calculated, quantitation of the severity of aortic insufficiency can be carried out, provided that there are no other significant valvular

F. 4.1. (A) Gradient echo (upper panels) and velocity phase contrast (lower panels) axial images in a patient with mild aortic regurgitation corresponding to systole (left panels) and diastole (right panels). The phase contrast image corresponding to diastole (right lower) does not show flow velocity signal in the encircled ascending aorta, as opposed to the systolic one (left lower), this indicating the absence of significant retrograde flow and, thus, the mild degree of aortic regurgitation. (B) Gradient echo (upper panels) and velocity phase contrast (lower panels) coronal images in systole (left panels) and diastole (right panels) in the same patient. The right superior panel shows a signal void phenomenon (arrow) corresponding to the mild aortic insufficiency.

F. 4.2. Flow curve at the level of the ascending aorta in a patient with severe aortic regurgitation. The presence of negative flow during diastole in the aorta can be detected, the relationship between positive systolic and negative diastolic flows allowing the calculation of the regurgitant volume and fraction of the regurgitation.

F. 4.3. (A) Axial spin echo showing prolapse of the posterior mitral leaflet (arrow). (B) Systolic gradient echo image of the same patient where a signal void effect due to a mitral regurgitant turbulent flow is seen (arrow) with a highly eccentric distribution in close relation with the atrial aspect of the anterior mitral leaflet.

insufficiencies or shunts, by calculating the regurgitant fraction obtained from the comparison of the stroke volume of the left and right ventricles ([LVSV-RVSV]/LVSV), where LVSV is stroke volume of the left ventricle, RVSV is the stroke volume of the right ventricle and LVSV-RVSV equals the volume of aortic regurgitation. This is an accurate method to quantify aortic regurgitation[6,7].

c. Evaluation of regurgitation with cine gradient echo

By this method, images of the outflow tract of the left ventricle and the ascending aorta in coronal planes of the thorax are obtained, from which the severity of aortic regurgitation can be evaluated as the turbulence and high flow velocity of the regurgitant jet appear in the image of cine gradient echo as an area of signal void that highly contrasts with the normal flow in the interior of the left ventricular chamber[8] (Figure 4.1B). The width, depth, and the area or the volume of the turbulent regurgitation jet are related to regurgitation severity similarly to the current echocardiographic color flow map techniques.

The acceleration of flow proximal to the regurgitant leak produces a diastolic signal void near the aortic side of the valve. Its size correlates with the grade of aortic regurgitation[9]. Another quantitative aproach to this method by velocity mapping has been proposed[10].

4.5 Mitral and Tricuspid Regurgitation

a. Quantitation with cine velocity mapping

Mitral insufficiency can be quantitated with this technique by calculation of flow volume in the mitral ring and ascending aorta[11]. The difference between left ventricular inflow volume and aortic flow volume, and the regurgitant fraction can be calculated in order to estimate the severity of mitral regurgitation.

Another approach to qualitative estimation of tricuspid insufficiency is based on the study of flow the vena cava. The flow of the superior vena cava can also be estimated on the same plane used to analyze the aorta (Figure 4.4). Flow can be calculated from data obtained from velocity maps by multiplying the area of the vena cava section during each cardiac cycle by its velocity. In normal subjects, a systolic and a diastolic wave toward the right atrium and another retrograde diastolic wave that coincides with atrial contraction are observed[12]. Patients with significant tricuspid regurgitation display a flat or inverted systolic wave (Figure 4.5).

b. Quantitation of regurgitant volume using Simpson's method

Volume calculation is carried out using the same method as the one described for aortic regurgitacion. Quantitation of the regurgitant fraction is obtained by comparing the stroke volume of the left and right ventricles ([LVSV-RVSV]/LVSV, where LVSV-RVSV equals the mitral regurgitant volume. This parameter has proved to have an excellent correlation with the severity of mitral insufficiency, as long as no other significant regurgitations or shunts are present[6,7]. The same procedure is used for tricuspid insufficiency ([RVSV-LVSV]/RVSV), where RVSV-LVSV is the tricuspid regurgitant volume.

c. Evaluation with cine gradient echo

Oblique planes including the longitudinal axial of the left ventricle are preferred to visualize the origin of systolic turbulence of mitral regurgitation (Figure 4.3B and 4.6). Volume, depth and the area of the signal void due to turbulence within the left atrium can be calculated based on multiple, contiguous slices in cine gradient echo. These parameters are directly related to the severity of the insufficiency. The size of signal void near the ventricular aspect of the valve (Figure 4.6) can be used for the estimation of mitral regurgitation.

4.6 Pulmonary Regurgitation

Volume quantitation of pulmonary insufficiency by MRI can be accomplished by any

FIGURE 4.4

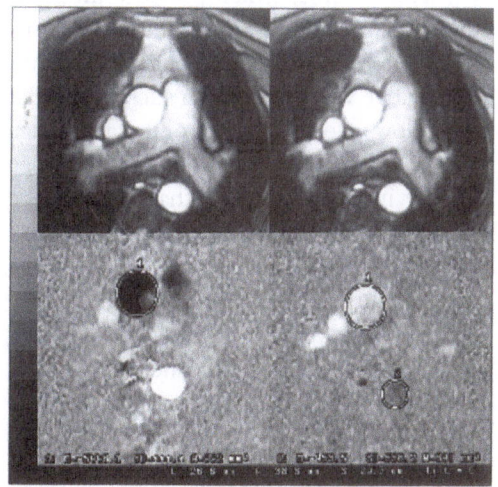

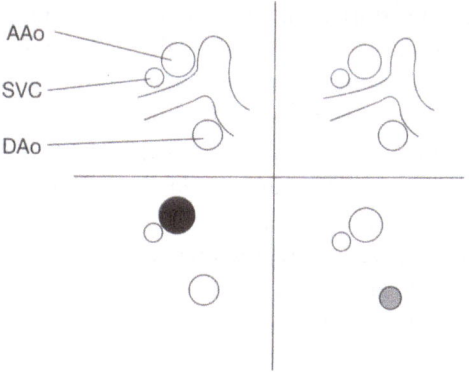

AAo

SVC

DAo

FIGURE 4.5

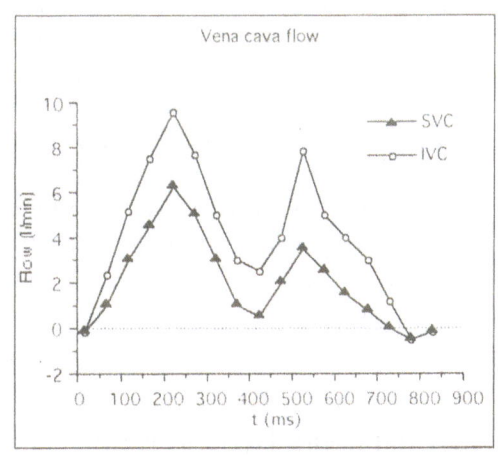

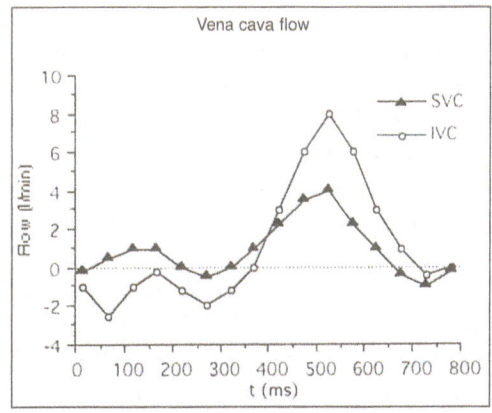

FIGURE 4.6

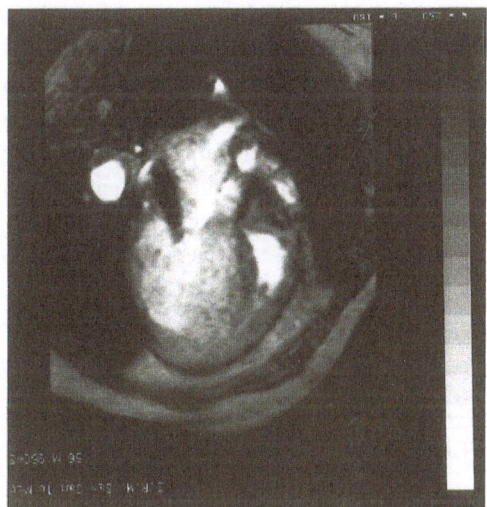

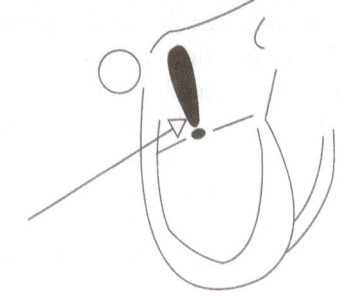

F. 4.4. Gradient echo (upper panels) and velocity phase contrast (lower panels) axial images in a patient with severe aortic regurgitation corresponding to systole (left panels) and diastole (right panels). Phase contrast images are encoded in this case in black for flow with a caudo-cranial direction and in white for the cranio-caudal direction. The left lower panel shows a normal systolic pattern of flow both at the level of the ascending and descending aorta. The right lower panel, instead, shows a bright grey pattern in the ascending aorta indicative of retrograde cranio-caudal flow due to the aortic regurgitation (compare with figure 4.1 A). AAo: ascending aorta; DAo: descending aorta; SVC: superior vena cava.

F. 4.5. Velocity maps of the superior and inferior vena cava. The upper graph corresponds to a normal individual, where both venae cavae exhibit well defined systolic and diastolic flow components. In the lower graph, which corresponds to a case of severe tricuspid insufficiency, the absence of systolic flow component in both venae cavae as a consequence of the increase in pressure secondary to tricuspid insufficiency can be noted.

F. 4.6. Systolic gradient echo image of a longitudinal plane of the heart. A signal void effect is noted in the left atrium, which corresponds to a moderate mitral insufficiency: note the area of proximal flow confluence on the ventricular asepct of the mitral valve (arrow).

of the previously described methods used for aortic insufficiency[13]. Regurgitant volume and regurgitant fraction calculation is carried out in the main pulmonary artery. The area below the diastolic curve of pulmonary flow corresponds to the pulmonary regurgitant flow. The regurgitant fraction is obtained from the division between the diastolic regurgitant volume and the ejection volume in systole.

4.7 Pulmonary Hypertension

MRI allows access to many aspects of the function and anatomy of the right cardiac chambers that reflect the consequences of pulmonary hypertension. Dilatation of the vena cava, right chambers and of the pulmonary arteries are findings related to pulmonary hypertension that are easily demonstrated with MRI. In these patients, anomalies in the pulsatile flow of the pulmonary arteries with patterns of flow with inversion at the end of systole and in diastole are found, as well as an early systolic velocity peak[14]. Pulmonary hypertension is calculated using methods similar to those used in Doppler echocardiography: the tricuspid regurgitation velocity is calculated in order to estimate the systolic gradient between the right ventricle and atrium and, when the estimated pressure in the right atrium is added to this gradient, systolic pulmonary pressure can be derived, as long as pulmonary stenosis is not present.

4.8 Valvular Stenosis

Valvular stenosis can be easily quantified by calculating the flow velocity, to which the simplified equation of Bernouilli is applied[15,16], as is done in the Doppler technique. The spatial and temporal profile of blood velocity can be recorded in images obtained on planes including the stenotic flow direction previously identified with cine gradient echo sequences.

The behavior of the stenotic jet can be registered in cine, which provides information similar to color Doppler, but with significant differences. MRI presents images with quantitative velocity maps in such a way that blood flow velocity at each point of the image can be determined, as well as the average velocity in a specific area, that can even be integrated in time. MRI maps can record velocities with practically no limits for the precise study of pathological hemodynamic gradients. Also, the possibility of analyzing the velocity in any spatial plane permits flow with any direction to be registered (Figure 4.7).

b. Cine gradient echo

In normal subjects, a bright white signal is registered during valvular opening, generated by physiological laminar flow. During valvular opening, and occasionally during its closure, transient turbulent signals that have no pathological significance may be recorded. Flow turbulence originated by valvular stenosis during opening is manifested as an area of signal void, represented in black in the cine gradient echo images. The spatial and temporal magnitude of the area of turbulence registered in the cine image is related to the severity of the stenosis. The irregularities of the calcified valvular leaflets contribute to the formation of turbulence and, on occasion, can magnify the signal void area in the cine image, with the result that the severity of the stenosis can be overestimated.

4.9 Prosthetic Valves

Although there is occasionally concern in submitting patients with cardiac valve prosthesis to an MRI evaluation, the examination is in fact not contraindicated (except in the case of some old valve prostheses). Instead, the technique can even be useful in the evaluation of the function of the prosthesis (Figure 4.8).

There are in vitro studies validating the measurements of transprosthetic flow velocity registered with this method[17]. The evaluation of the dysfunction of the valvular prosthesis has an excellent correlation with transesophageal echocardiography (TEE)[18].

FIGURE 4.7

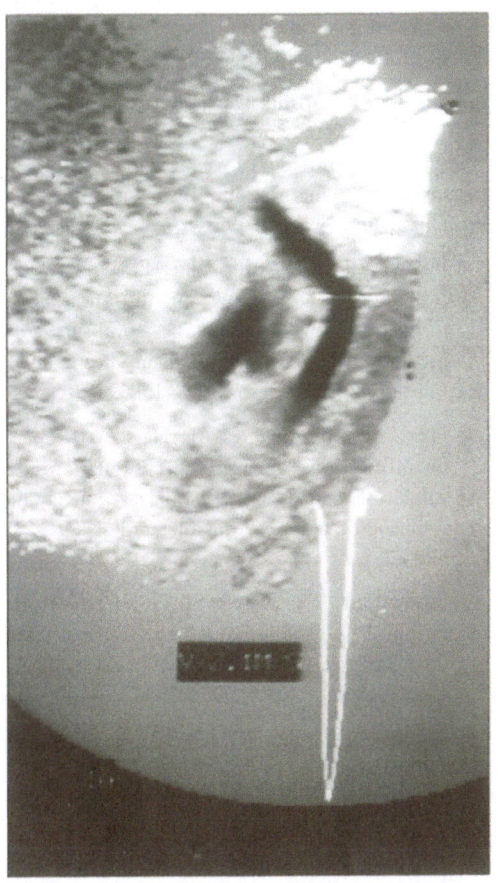

FIGURE 4.8

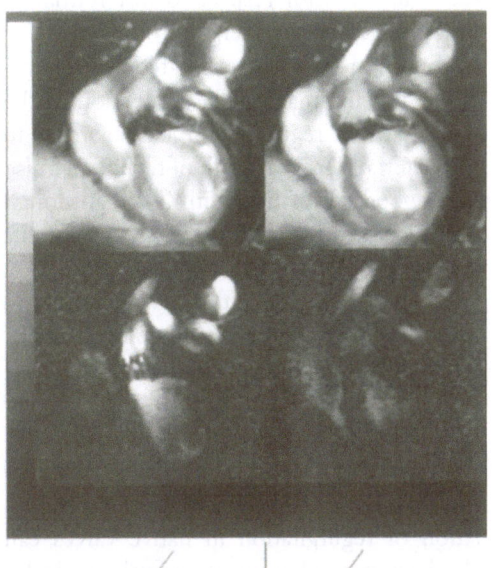

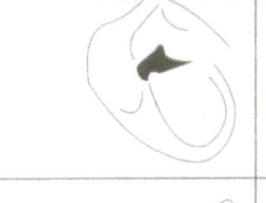 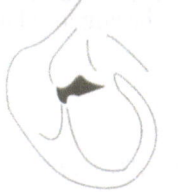

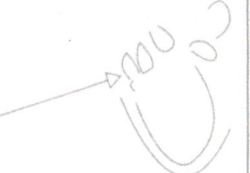 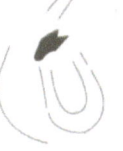

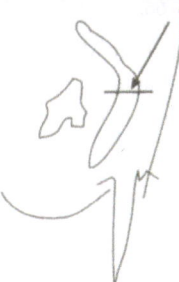

F. 4.7.   Biological pulmonary prosthesis: map and velocity curve showing a peak value of 2.1 m/s, obtained from a plane perpendicular to the transprosthetic flow (arrow).

F. 4.8.   Gradient echo (upper panels) and velocity phase contrast (lower panels) coronal images in a patient with a bileaflet mechanical aortic valve prosthesis corresponding to systole (left panels) and diastole (right panels). A small artifactual signal due to the prosthesis can be seen on the gradient echo images. The left lower panel shows the presence of two separate bright signals corresponding to the transprosthetic ejection flow (arrow); no flow signals are seen at the ventricular aspect of the prosthesis in diastole (right lower panel), this ruling out significant regurgitation.

The intra- or paraprosthetic origin of regurgitation with respect to differentiating physiological insufficiency from prosthetic dysfunction can be evaluated with cine gradient echo images. The evaluation of the severity of the regurgitation jets according to the criteria of area or depth of turbulence also has a good correlation with TEE. Although TEE is still the technique of choice for the study of these patients, MRI represents a valid alternative for patients who refuse to undergo transesophageal exploration or when diagnostic limitations occur.

Transprosthetic gradient during valvular opening can be determined by means of velocity maps (Figure 4.7), and quantitative methods previously described for the calculation of regurgitation in native valves can also be employed in the case of valvular leaks.

References

1. Jiménez-Borreguero LJ, Kilner PJ, Firmin DN. Precision of magnetic resonance velocity mapping to calculate flow: an in vitro study. J Cardiovasc Magn Reson 1998; 1: 85.

2. Caduff JH, Hernandez RJ, Ludomirsky A. MR visualization of aortic vegetations. J Comput Assist Tomogr 1996; 20: 613–5.

3. Akins EW, Limacher M, Slone RM, Hill JA. Evaluation of an aortic annular pseudoaneurysm by MRI: comparison with echocardiography, angiography and surgery. Cardiovasc Intervent Radiol 1987; 10: 188–93.

4. Manzara CC, Underwood SR, Pennell DJ, et al. Magnetic resonance velocity mapping for measurement of valvular regurgitation. Eur Heart J 1991; 12: 1786.

5. Dulce MC, Mostbeck GH, Friese KK, Caputo GR, Higgins CB. Quantification of the left ventricular volumes and function with cine MR imaging: comparison of geometric models with three-dimensional data. Radiology 1993; 188: 371–6.

6. Underwood SR, Klipstein RH, Firmin DN, et al. Magnetic resonance assessment of aortic and mitral regurgitation. Br Heart J 1986; 56: 455–62.

7. Sechtem U, Pflugfelder PW, Cassidy MM, et al. Mitral or aortic regurgitation: Quantification of regurgitant volumes with cine MR imaging. Radiology 1988; 167: 425–30.

8. Higgins CB, Wagner S, Kondo C, Suzuki J, Caputo GR. Evaluation of valvular heart disease with cine gradient echo magnetic resonance imaging. Circulation 1991; 84(3 Suppl.): I198–207.

9. Yoshida K, Yoshikawa J, Hozmi T, et al. Assessment of aortic regurgitation by the acceleration flow signal void proximal to the leak orifice in cinemagnetic resonance imaging. Circulation 1991; 83: 1951–5.

10. Jimenez-Borreguero LJ, Kilner PJ, Underwood SR, Firmin DN. Flow quantification with magnetic resonance using the isovelocity area method close to an orifice: an in vitro study. J Cardiovasc Magn Reson 1998; 1: 85.

11. Fujita N, Chazouilleres AF, Hartiala JJ, et al. Quantification of mitral regurgitation by velocity-encoded cine nuclear magnetic resonance imaging. J Am Coll Cardiol 1994; 23: 951–8.

12. Mohiaddin RH, Wann SL, Underwood R, Firmin DN, Rees S, Longmore DB. Vena caval flow: assessment with cine MR velocity mapping. Radiology 1990; 177: 537–41.

13. Rebergen SA, Chin JG, Ottenkamp J, van der Wall EE, de Roos A. Pulmonary regurgitation in the late postoperative follow-up of tetralogy of Fallot. Volumetric quantitation by nuclear magnetic resonance velocity mapping. Circulation 1993; 88: 2257–66.

14. Kondo C, Caputo GR, Masui T, et al. Pulmonary hypertension: Pulmonary flow quantification and flow profile analysis with velocity-encoded cine MR imaging. Radiology 1992; 183: 751.

15. Kilner PJ, Manzara CC, Mohiaddin RH, et al. Magnetic resonance jet velocity mapping in mitral and aortic valve stenosis. Circulation 1993; 87: 1239–48.

16. Kilner PJ, Firmin DN, Rees RS, et al. Valve and great vessel stenosis: assessment with MR jet velocity mapping. Radiology 1991; 178: 229–35.

17. Walker PG, Pedersen EM, Oyre S, et al. Magnetic resonance velocity imaging: a new method for prosthetic heart valve study. J Heart Valve Dis 1995; 4: 296–307.

18. Deutsch HJ, Bachmann R, Sechtem U, et al. Regurgitant flow in cardiac valve prostheses: diagnostic value of gradient echo nuclear magnetic resonance imaging in reference to transesophageal two-dimensional color Doppler echocardiography. J Am Coll Cardiol 1992; 19: 1500–7.

Magnetic resonance imaging of ischemic heart disease

5

F. CARRERAS-COSTA

5.1   Introduction

MRI offers a comprehensive morphological and functional evaluation of the heart[1] and coronary vessels[2], because of its soft tissue contrast capabilities, allowing the characterization of myocardial tissue[3], and providing an excellent spatial and temporal resolution as well as the potential for three-dimensional studies[4]. Thus, MRI has a promising future with respect to the care of patients with ischemic heart disease, and will compete advantageously with other cardiac imaging techniques[5].

The tomographic and multiplanar imaging capabilities and the ability to perform cine MRI sequences in any spatial plane allow the identification of ventricular endocardial and epicardial contours and the accurate assessment of left ventricular mass and volume as well as the determination of systolic wall thickening and regional wall motion abnormalities[6]. Spin echo images allow the identification of the scar of a chronic myocardial infarction, due to the thinning of the myocardial wall[7] (Figure 5.1), whereas dynamic studies to assess cardiac function and perfusion are possible under pharmacologic stress conditions[8]. Image resolution is superior to echocardiography and it does not have its artifact limitations.

MRI permits reliable and reproducible measurements of left ventricular volumes and mass without any geometrical hypothesis, and so remain valid in presence of ventricular deformation as observed after a myocardial infarction[9]. This requires the application of Simpson's rule, that adds the myocardial volume directly calculated from each contiguous transverse slice covering the whole left ventricle, as explained in chapter 2. An exact and reproducible calculation of left ventricular mass and volume in patients who have suffered a myocardial infarction may be of great interest in the longitudinal follow-up studies of myocardial remodeling, as it permits the study of the changes secondary to therapeutic intervention[10].

5.2   Acute Myocardial Infarction

The alterations produced by the presence of myocardial edema after infarction in the myocardial relaxation times allow the direct identification of an acute myocardial infarction[11] in the spin echo T2 weighted MR images (Figure 5.2). Nevertheless, the frequently suboptimal quality of the image, degraded by the low signal-to-noise ratio of T2 weighted sequences, does not permit a high diagnostic sensitivity. The use of quelated paramagnetic extracellular contrast agents[12], such as gadolinium-diethylenetri-aminepenta-acetic acid (Gd-DTPA), allows the detection with enhanced resolution of the heterogeneity of regional myocardial perfusion during an acute ischemic injury, and makes possible the identification and quantitation of areas of acute or subacute myocardial necrosis in T1 weighted spin echo and gradient echo sequences[13] (Figure 5.3), as explained in chapter 9.

MRI can also be used as a comprehensive examination in patients with infarction, assessing in the same study such different parameters as left ventricular structure, global and regional function, infarct artery patency (see later) and contrast uptake[14].

5.3   Complications of Myocardial Infarction

a. Ventricular aneurysm
Spin echo and gradient echo techniques are useful for the identification of ventricular aneurysms and the delimitation of their extension (Figure 5.4 and 5.5), aiding in the surgical decision as well as in its technical planning. The ability of MRI to reproduce the same slice planes in serial studies improves the accuracy in the assessment of the anatomical changes after surgical correction (Figures 5.6 and 5.7).

The noninvasive character of MRI and its high resolution to image paracardiac structures, as opposed to echocardiography,

makes easier the diagnosis of the hemo-pericardium effusion secondary to a subacute left ventricular free-wall rupture (Figure 5.8), which may later evolve into the formation of a ventricular pseudoaneurysm (Figure 5.9).

c. Intraventricular thrombosis
Although intraventricular thrombus can be identified with static spin echo T1 images (Figure 5.10), diagnostic doubts may exist when flow artifacts are present in cases of aneurysmal ventricular dilatation and blood stagnation. It is useful then to perform a cine MRI sequence using the gradient echo technique, which makes it possible to easily differentiate between a flow artifact and an organized thrombus[15] (Figure 5.11).

d. Mitral regurgitation
Although MRI is not the technique of choice for the diagnosis of mitral insufficiency, it is possible to identify its presence by means of cine MRI (Figure 5.12), as has been mentioned in chapter 4.

5.4   Study of Ventricular Function

MRI has proven to be an effective, exact and reproducible technique to determine the measurements and functional parameters of both ventricles[16]. Cine MRI sequences obtained by gradient echo techniques display the myocardial wall borders with a good temporal resolution (16 to 30 images per cardiac cycle) and without interferences. The motion sensitivity of cardiac MRI can be exploited to measure the motion patterns within the heart wall and thus noninvasively calculate the intramyocardial strain[17].

a. Global ventricular function
When segmental alterations of contractily are present, in order to perform rapid calculation of the ejection fraction it is necessary to use the biplane method, which requires two and four-chamber planes (Figure 5.13). A more exact method, but time consuming, is the direct calculation of systolic and diastolic volumes using Simpson's method, from consecutive transverse sections of the left ventricle

FIGURE 5.1 A and B

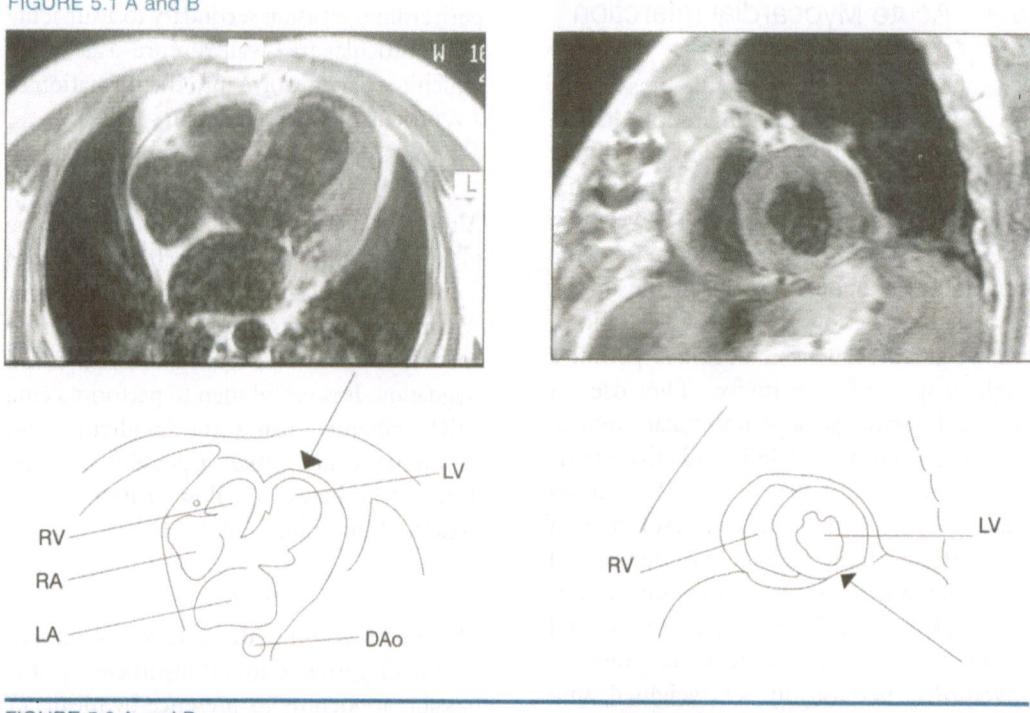

FIGURE 5.2 A and B

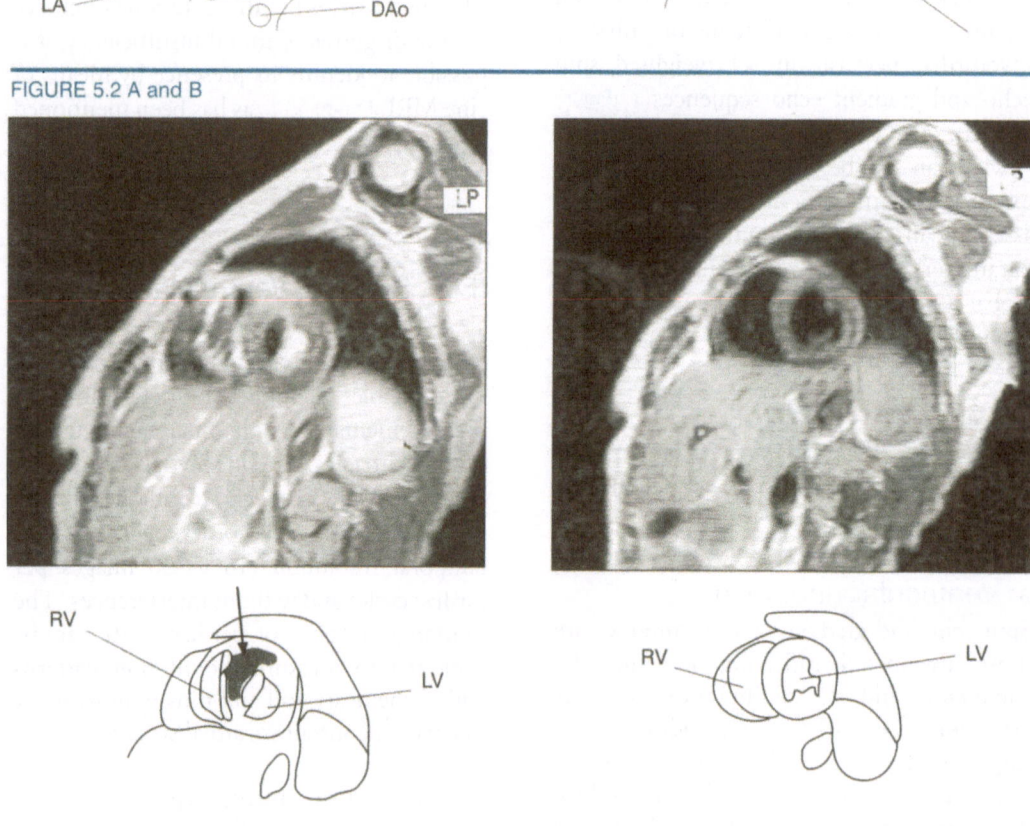

F. 5.1　(A) T1 spin echo diastolic image of the cardiac chambers in the axial plane. A marked reduction of the left ventricular wall thickness at the left ventricular antero-septal and apical segments is observed (arrow), characteristic of chronic myocardial necrosis in the region supplied by the left anterior descending coronary artery. (B) Ventricular short axis view in systole obtained by a sagittal oblique T1 spin echo plane; the absent contraction of the posterior left ventricular myocardial wall identifies an area of chronic necrosis (arrow). DAo: descending aorta; LA: left atrium; LV: left ventricle; RA: right atrium; RV: right ventricle.

F. 5.2.　Left ventricular short axis obtained during the subacute phase of an antero-septal myocardial infarction. In the T2 weighted spin echo image (A), an area of high signal intensity is observed in the anterior septum (arrow), caused by tissue edema in the infarcted region. No differential signal intensity changes are detected in a T1 weighted spin echo sequence obtained in the same patient and with the same orientation (B). LV: left ventricle; RV: right ventricle.

FIGURE 5.3 A and B

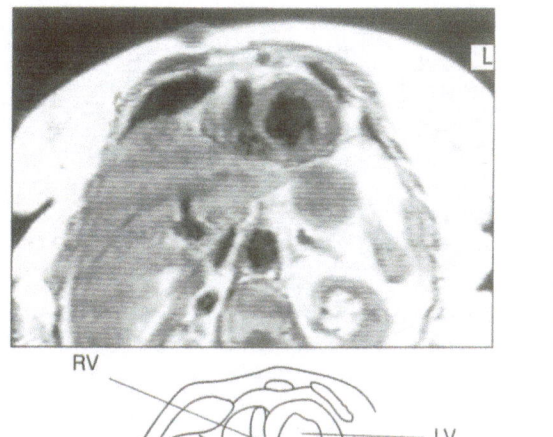
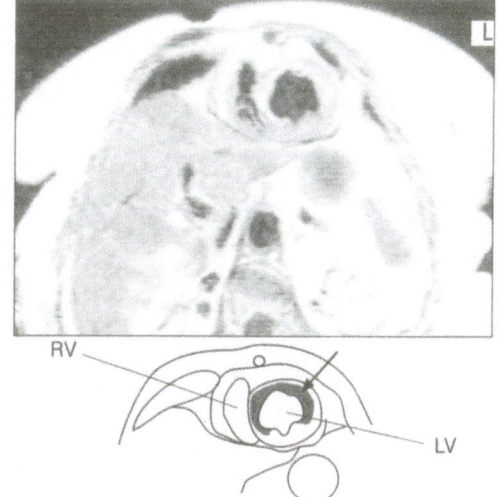

FIGURE 5.4

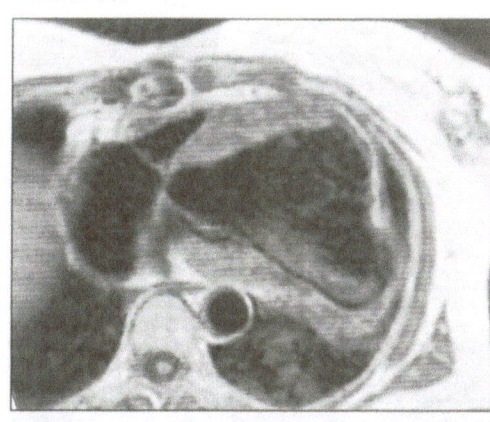
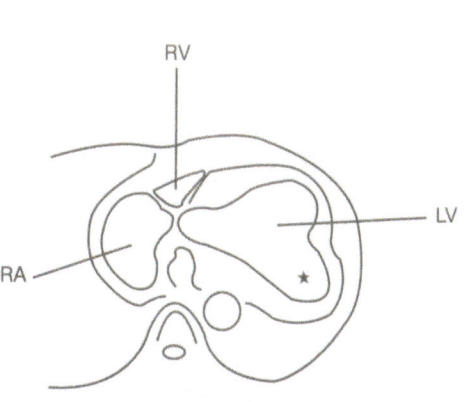

FIGURE 5.5 A and B

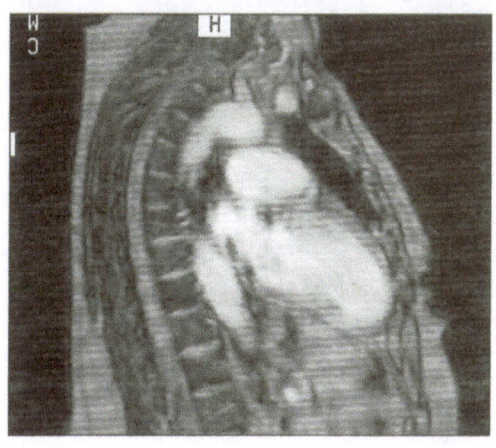
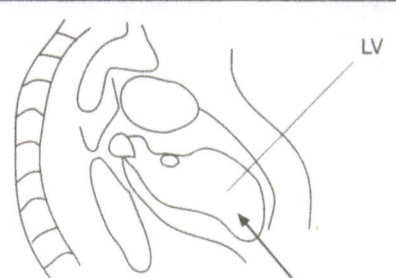
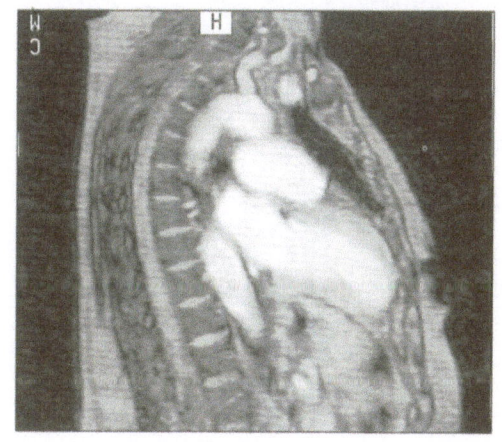
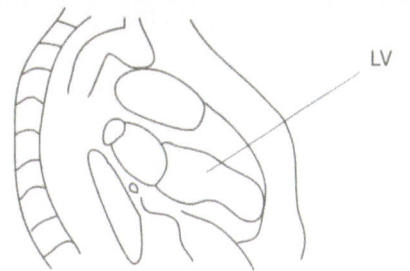

FIGURE 5.6 A and B

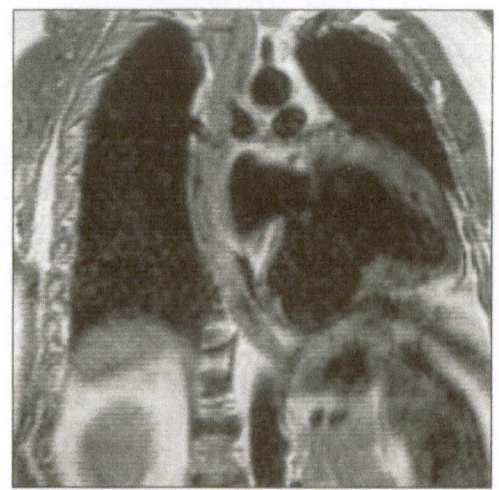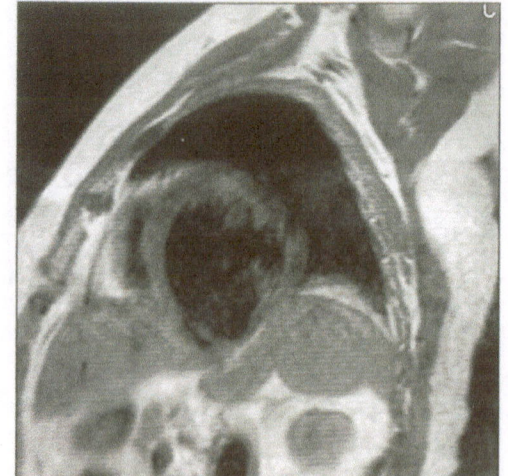

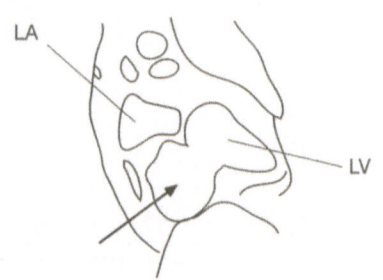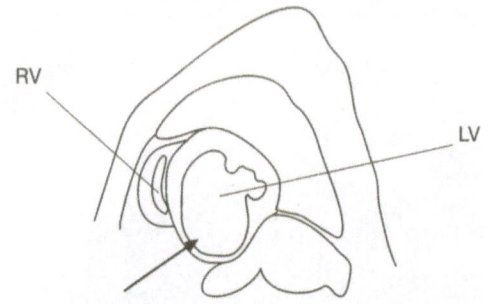

FIGURE 5.7 A and B

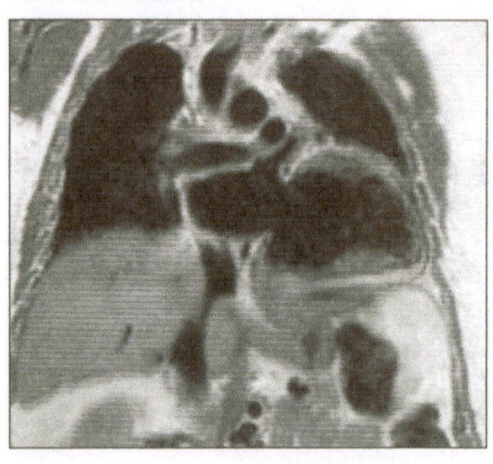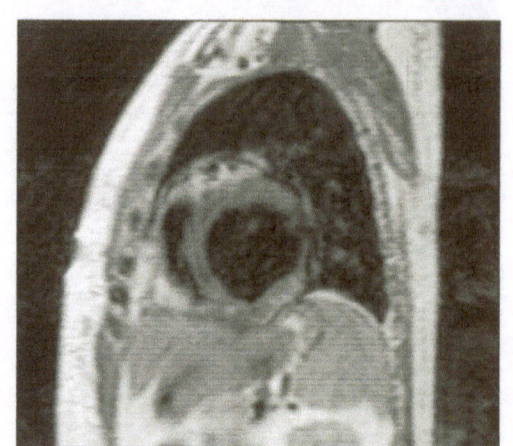

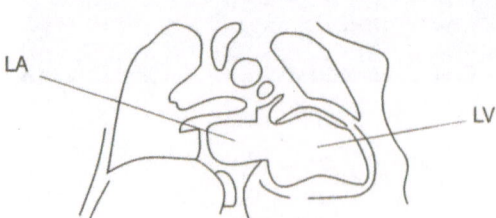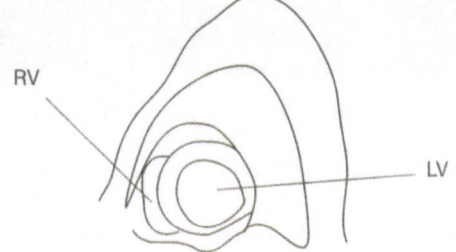

obtained in a multiplane-multiphase sequence. Both methods are very reproducible due to the high resolution of the MR images[18]. MRI has also proven to be a suitable technique to measure the volume and mass of the right ventricle[19], a structure which, due to its anatomical irregularities, requires the use of Simpson's rule.

b. Regional ventricular function

In order to measure the changes in systolic thickening of the left ventricular wall, it is necessary to analyze the end-diastolic and end-systolic frames of a cine MRI sequence, or the corresponding triggered-ECG spin echo still images, of a left ventricular short axis (Figure 5.14). However, conventional sequences are time consuming for the acquisition and analysis of these images. Innovative equipment now permits imaging time of cine MRI to be shortened considerably by using rapid sequences. At the same time, software analysis for left ventricular endocardial border detection is being developed, with the aim of permitting the automated analysis of the left ventricular radial contractility and the regional variations of systolic thickening[20]. This software is currently available, but the main difficulty lies in the design of appropriate algorithms for the automated recognition of borders. A practical alternative option would be the use of commercial available software designed for echocardiographic analysis to perform off-line measurements of MRI information.

Methods for the noninvasive measurement of three-dimensional myocardial motion with MRI have recently been developed using presaturation tagging and velocity-encoded phase maps. The combination of breath-hold imaging with tagging and velocity-encoded sequences has made the measurement of myocardial wall motion a reproducible examination, permitting the quantification of the severity and extent of regional heart wall motion abnormalities both at rest and during stress[21].

c. Evaluation under pharmacological stress

The technical impossibility of obtaining appropriate MRI images during exercise turns the study of regional and global left ventricular contractile function under pharmacological stimulation into a technique of great interest for the detection of myocardial ischemia[22]. The reduction or absence of systolic myocardial thickening is the first functional marker of ischemia, which manifests itself even before electro-cardiographic alterations[23]. Published studies refer to the use of dipyridamole[24] and dobutamine[25,26], with an administration protocol similar to that which is normally used in echocardiographic studies. The only technical requisite is that cardiac frequency should be stable during image acquisition. Likewise, it is advisable to maintain continuous communication with the patient during the examination, in order to evaluate the appearance of symptoms during the study. If they are available, it is recommended to use cine-MRI turbo-flash sequences, with a shorter duration than those obtained by gradient echo, and with a suitable image resolution to permit the application of software programs for the quantitative analysis of thickening and segmental left ventricular contractility. Although the images obtained by MRI have a very good resolution with respect to echocardiography, the inconvenience is, at least at the present, that a complete study of segmental wall function is a time-consuming process.

F. 5.3. Left ventricular short axis plane obtained during the subacute phase of a large antero-septal myocardial infarction. (A) Basal image. (B) Image obtained 20 minutes following adminstration of Gd-DTPA paramagnetic contrast; while the contrast has been completely washed from the myocardial segments with normal perfusion, the infarcted antero-septal segment shows increased signal intensity due to the delayed wash-in and wash-out of Gd-DTPA. RV: right ventricle; LV: left ventricle.

F. 5.4. Axial plane at the level of the cardiac chambers: a large postero-lateral ventricular aneurysm is observed (asterisk). LV: left ventricle; RV: right ventricle.

F. 5.5. Diastolic (A) and systolic (B) images of a cine-MRI sequence in a case of apical left ventricular aneurysm. LV: left ventricle.

F. 5.6 Ventricular aneurysm located at the infero-basal wall visualized in the longitudinal (A) and transverse (B) planes of the left ventricle. Note the indentation on the diaphragm caused by the aneurysm. LA: left atrium; LV: left ventricle.

F. 5.7. Images from the same patient as in figure 5.5 and with the same orientation (A and B), following surgical resection of the aneurysm. LA: left atrium; LV: left ventricle.

FIGURE 5.8

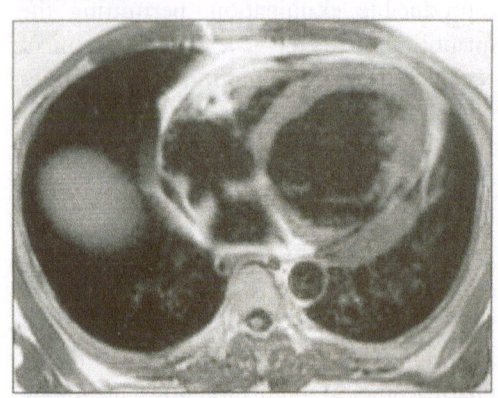
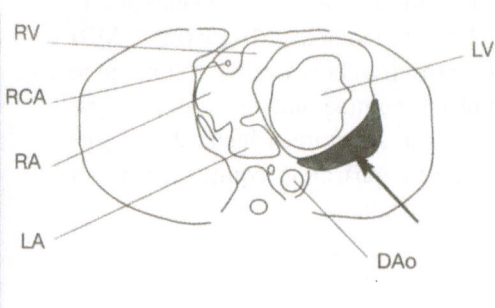

FIGURE 5.9 A, B and C

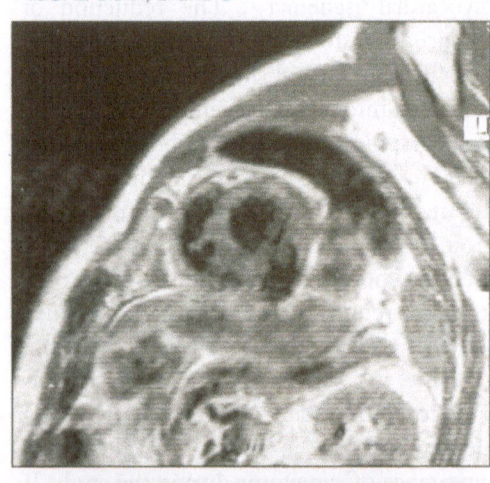
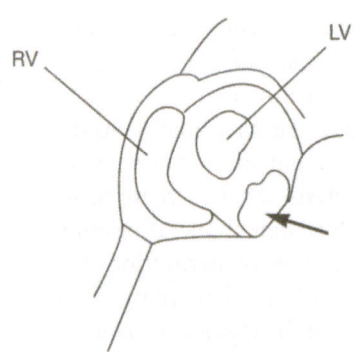

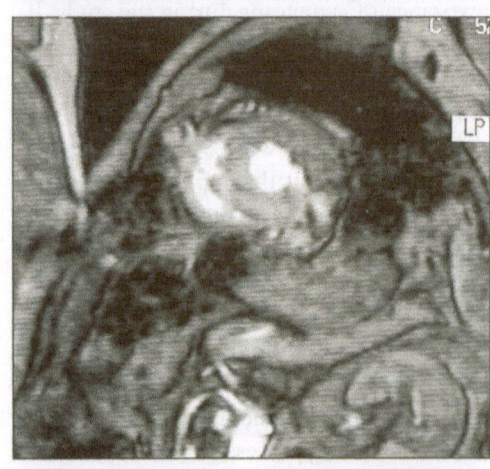
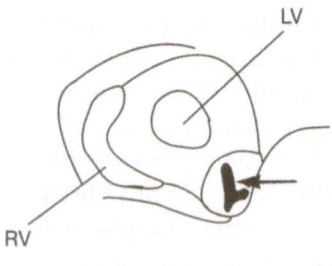

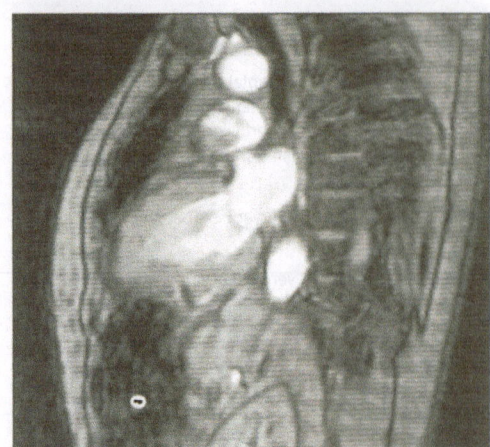
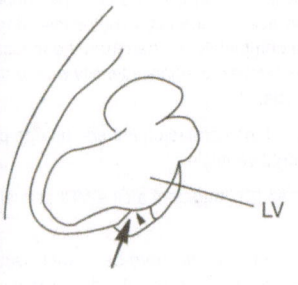

FIGURE 5.10

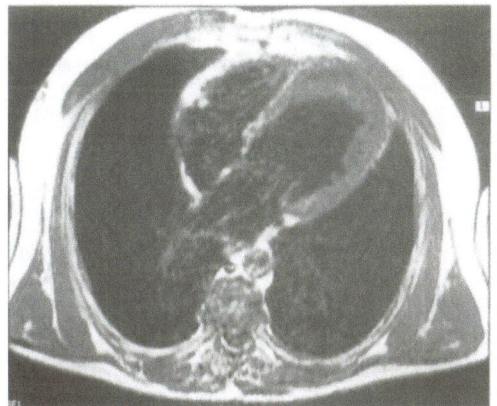

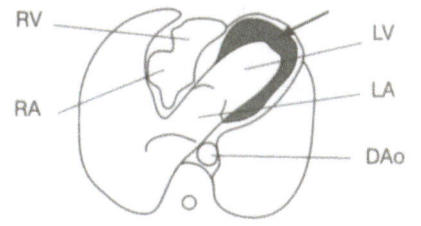

FIGURE 5.12

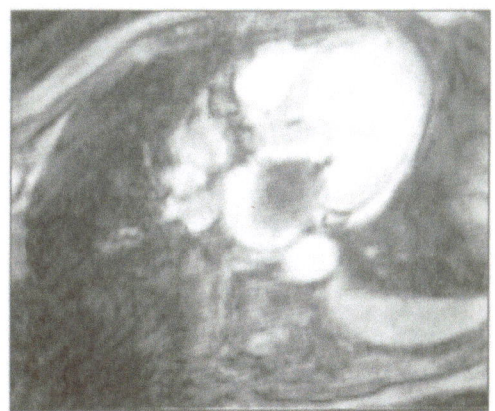

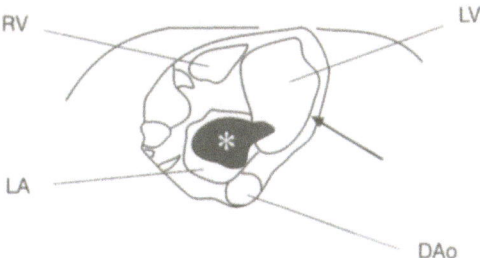

F. 5.8. Axial image of the left ventricle, where a marked thinning of the posterior ventricular wall may be observed, with a localized and contained pericardial effusion proven to be secondary to an anfractuous subacute rupture of the infarcted myocardium later at surgery. This condition can be viewed as the first step in the formation of a pseudoaneurysm. DAo: descending aorta; LA: left atrium; LV: left ventricle; RA: right atrium; RCA: coronary artery; RV: right ventricle.

F. 5.9. Left ventricular postinfarction pseudoaneurysm. (A) T1 spin echo short axis view of the left ventricle showing the image of an apparent cavity (arrow) probably connected with the left ventricle through a rupture in the left ventricular wall; note the absence of identifiable myocardial wall signal in the external wall of this cavity. (B) Systolic image from a cine MRI gradient echo sequence with the same orientation showing a flow signal of a turbulent jet (arrow) entering the psedoaneurysmal cavity from the true left ventricle. (C) Systolic frame of a cine MRI sequence oriented on a longitudinal view of the left ventricle exhibiting the same finding (arrow).

F. 5.10. T1 spin echo image of an intraventricular laminar thrombus located into an apical aneurysm of the left ventricle. DAo: descending aorta; LA: left atrium; LV: left ventricle; RA: right atrium; RV: right ventricle.

FIGURE 5.11

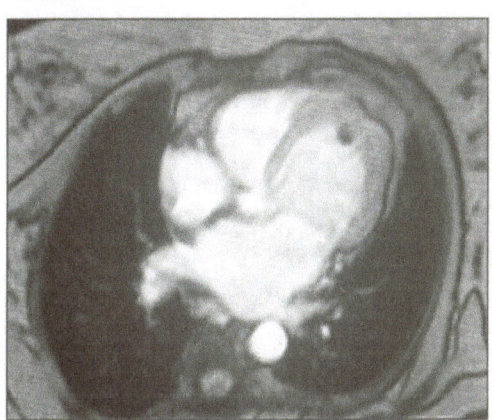

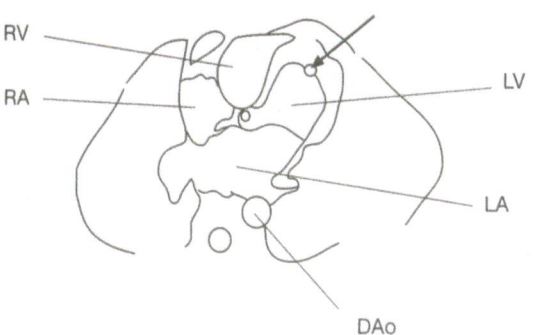

F. 5.11. Image of a cine MRI gradient echo sequence of an apical thrombus. DAo: descending aorta; LA: left atrium; LV: left ventricle; RA: right atrium; RV: right ventricle.

Systolic frame of a cine MRI sequence in which a left atrial signal void produced by an ischemic mitral regurgitation is seen (arrow). Note the absence of systolic thickening of the left ventricular lateral wall due to a previous infarction. DAo: descending aorta; LA: left atrium; LV: left ventricle; RV: right ventricle.

FIGURE 5.13 A and B

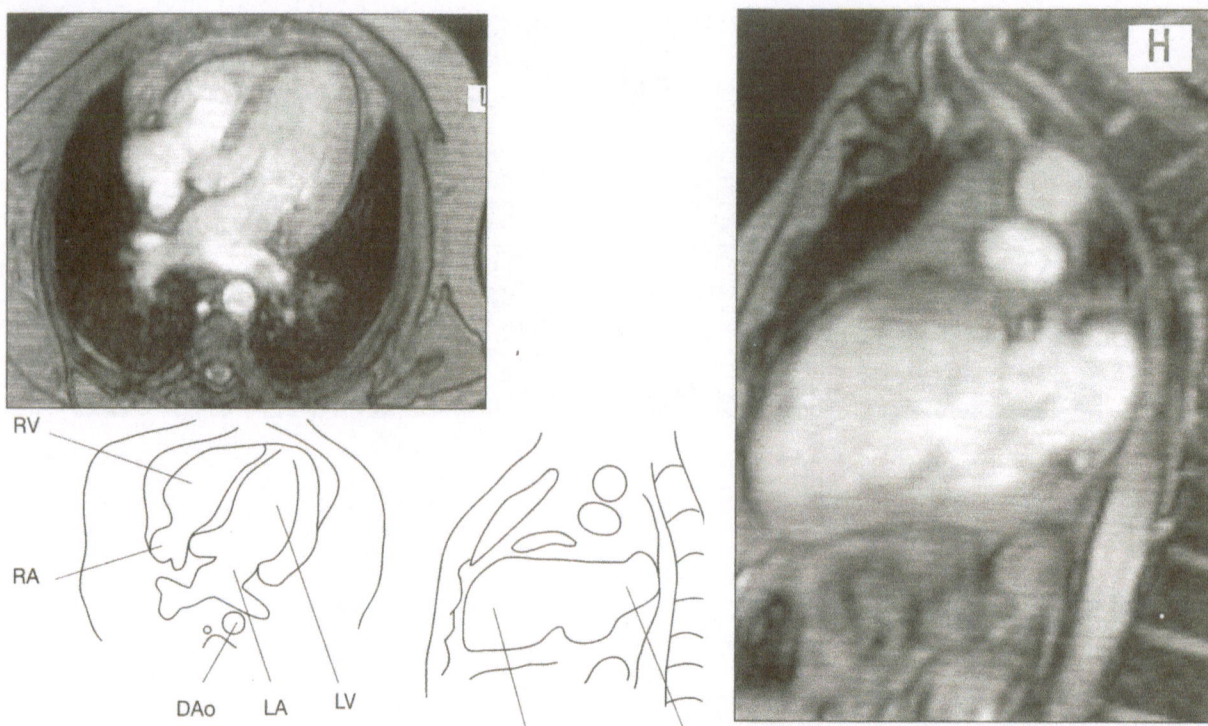

FIGURE 5.14 A and B

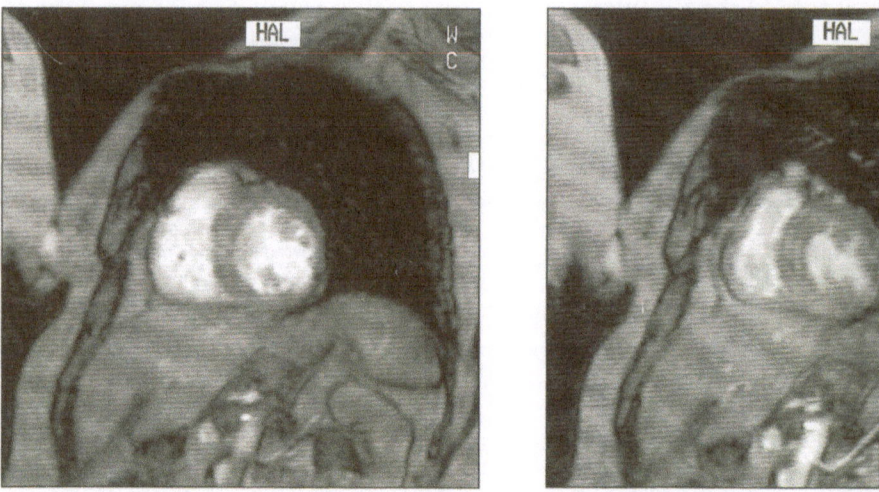

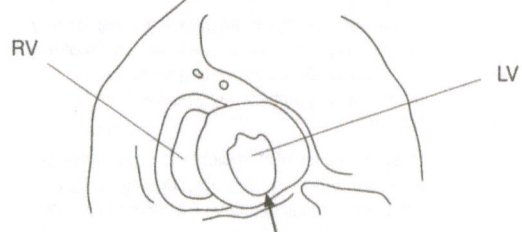

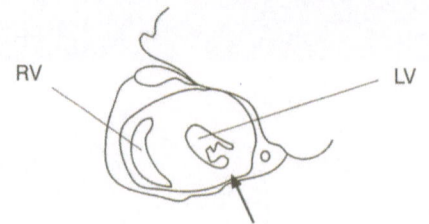

5.5 Imaging of Coronary Arteries

Despite the optimistic preliminary results published[27,28], predicting a promising future for MRI as the first noninvasive technique able to visualize the coronary artery anatomy, technical problems still persist preventing its use in clinical practice[29]. Nevertheless, new improvements in MRI hardware and software technology can offer impressive 3D images of the coronary tree[30], bringing close the time when coronary MRI studies will be routine.

The left coronary artery can usually be identified using conventional spin echo T1 images (Figure 5.15). Nevertheless, it is not an adequate method to detect the presence of stenotic lesions, since the prolonged signal acquisition time allows the respiratory movements to interfere with the image of the vessels. The development of rapid sequences using the breath-hold segmental-k-space gradient echo techniques has been the key factor to image the coronary arteries. This acquisition program permits a high resolution image to be obtained in 15–20 seconds, a time lapse during which the patients can hold their breath. In this way it is possible to obtain an image without respiratory movement artifacts, and the coronary vessels are visualized with greater definition and similar characteristics to those obtained by conventional gradient echo imaging. A particular characteristic of breath-hold sequences is that they contain a fat-suppression algorithm, eliminating the intense bright fat signal that can shade the view of the coronary vessel lumen. In spite of these technical improvements, the images that are obtained in practice with the current techniques are limited to the first two thirds length of the epicardial coronary vessels (Figure 5.16). The epicardial segment of the right coronary artery course is the easiest to visualize. The fact that the images are obtained in a 2D plane makes it difficult to encompass a long segment of the vessel in one single image (Figure 5.17). Three-dimensional reconstruction will make easier the recognition and analysis of the coronary vessel tree. Currently, a maximum spatial resolution of 1 mm can be obtained, while it is three times higher in coronary angiography. Therefore, it is still not possible to visualize stenotic coronary lesions with adequate resolution[31]. On the other hand, flow velocity assessment by means of MR phase velocity mapping sequences is an alternative method for the evaluation of vessel patency. Currently described applications of this technique could be the detection of an open artery after an acute myocardial infarction[32], or the evaluation of coronary artery bypass graft patency, whether they are saphenous vein grafts (Figures 5.18–5.20) or internal mammary artery grafts[33] (Figure 5.21). It should be kept in mind that the identification of a coronary vessel or a bypass graft depends on the presence of flowing blood in its lumen, since this is the target of MRI techniques, producing the typical black blood flow signal in spin echo imaging or an intense bright blood flow signal in gradient echo imaging. In a good quality image, the lack of recognition of a bypass graft in its expected place would predict its occlusion.

MRI is thus a technique with an extraordinary potential for the study of ischemic heart disease, due to the broad spectrum of information it can provide and to its non-invasive nature. At present, cardiac MRI is undergoing a period of rapid technical development, a process that is favored by the increasing number of cardiologists who are interested in its application. An important feature of the technique is that it permits the complete evaluation of the patient suffering ischemic heart disease[34,35], with the analysis under basal conditions and after pharmacological stress of global and segmental contractility and of myocardial perfusion.

F. 5.13. Cine MRI frames showing a four-chamber (A) and two-chamber (B) orthogonal longitudinal planes of the left ventricle. The first orientation allows the study of the contractile function of the septal and lateral walls, while that of the anterior and inferior segments is better evaluated in the two-chamber view. DAo: descending aorta; LA: left atrium; LV: left ventricle; RA: right atrium; RV: right ventricle.

F. 5.14. End-diastolic (A) and end-systolic (B) images from a patient with an old postero-lateral necrosis showing lack of systolic thickening in this segment (arrow). LV: left ventricle; RV: right ventricle.

FIGURE 5.15 A and B

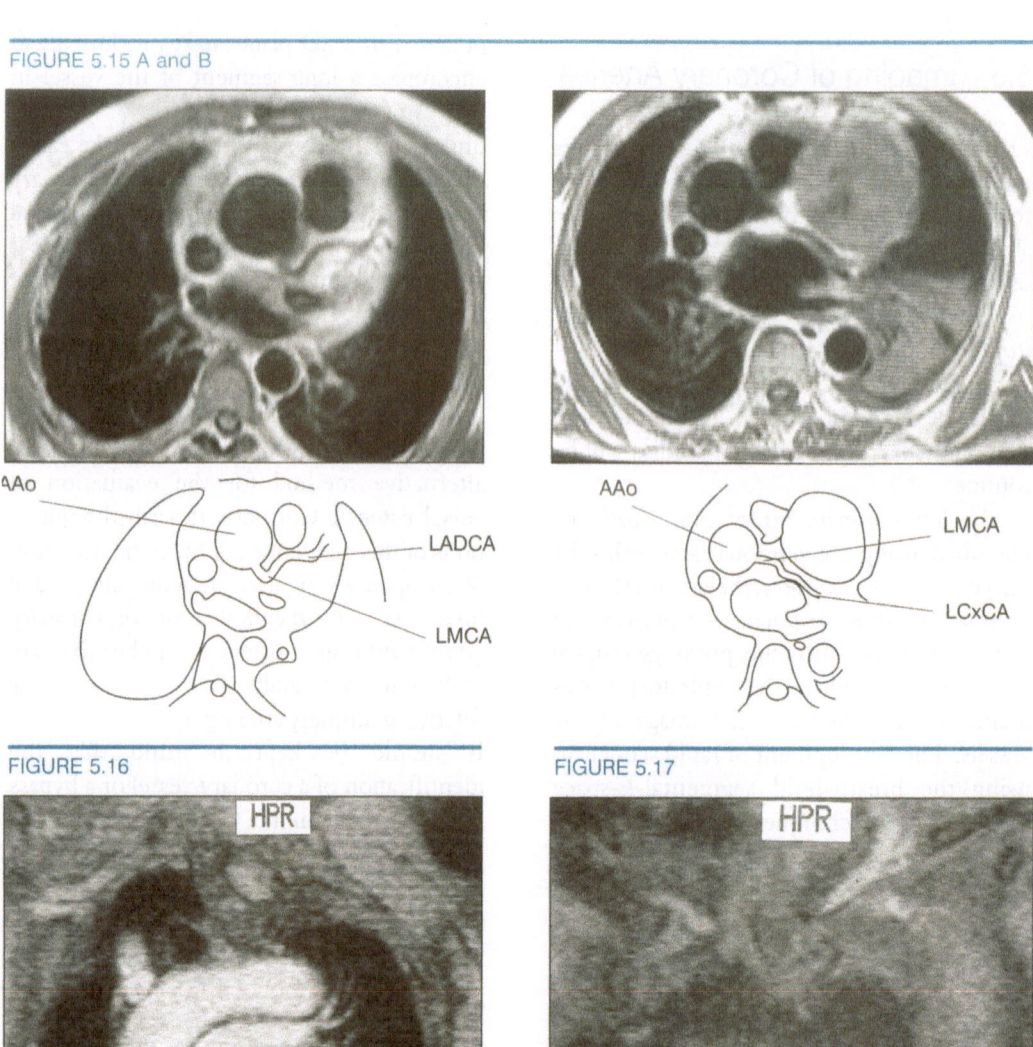

FIGURE 5.16

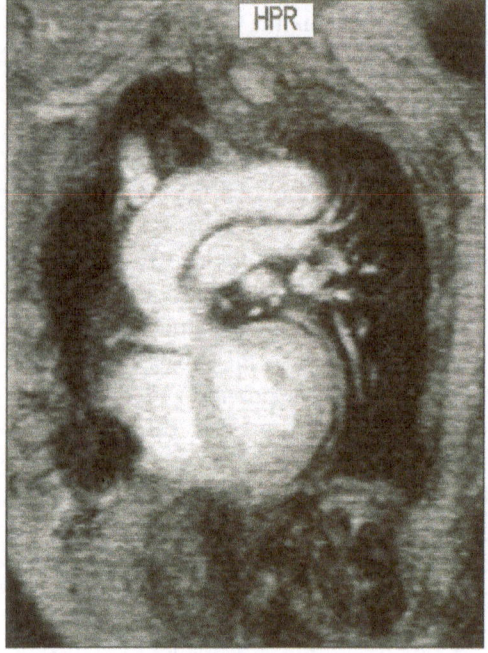

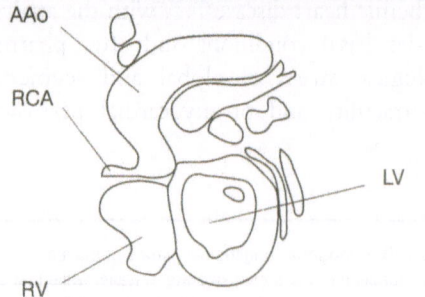

FIGURE 5.17

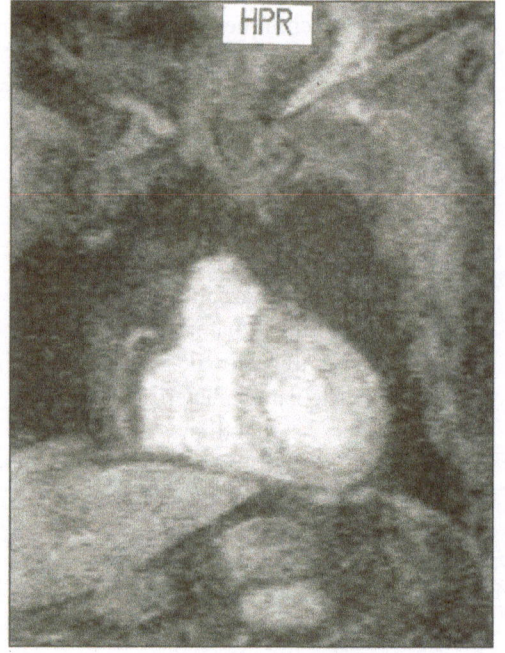

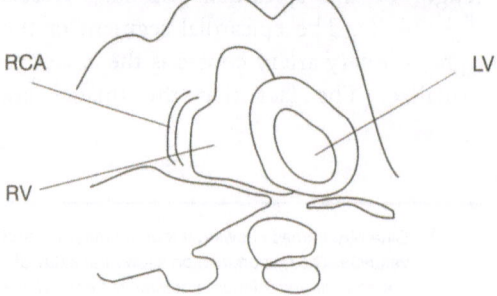

FIGURE 5.18 A and B

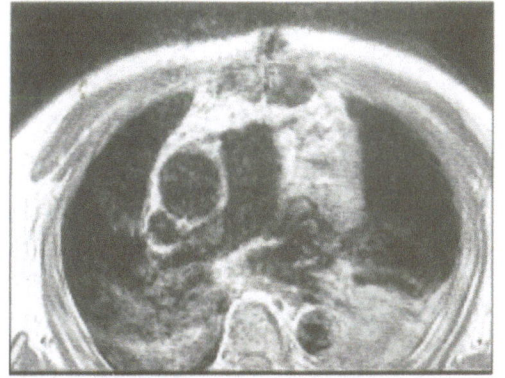

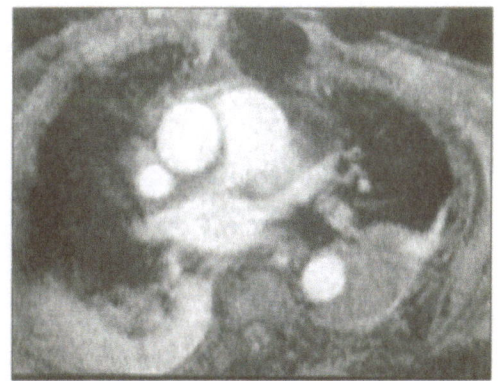

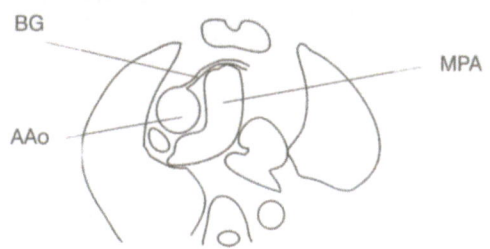

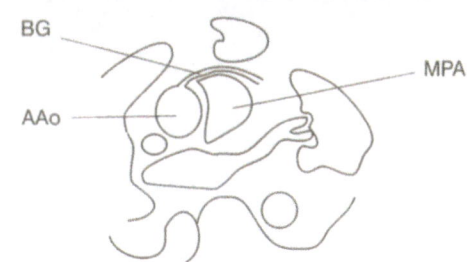

FIGURE 5.19

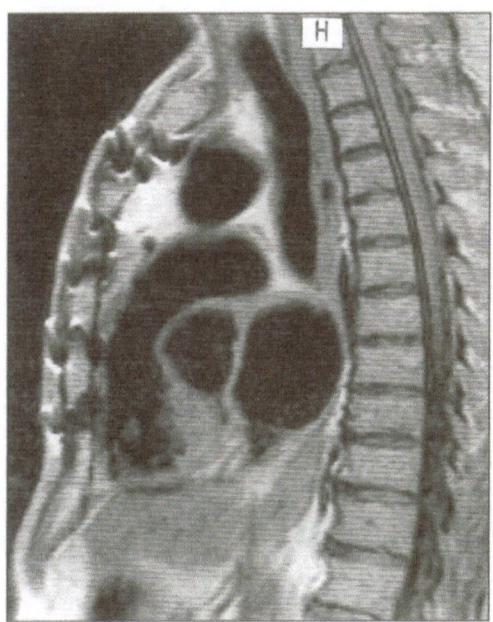

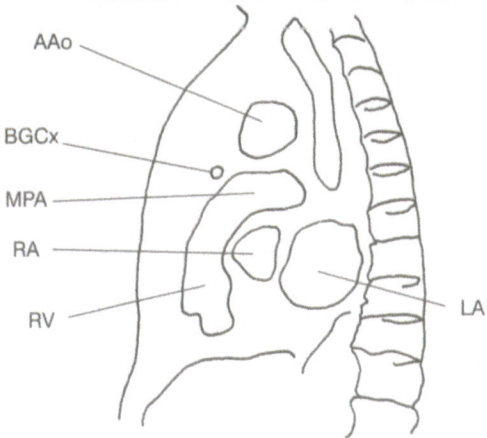

F. 5.15. Images of two consecutive spin echo T1 axial planes where the left coronary artery is depicted. In (A) the main left and left anterior descending coronary artery are identified (arrow). In (B) the circumflex artery, located on a lower spatial plane, is observed (arrow). AAo: Ascending aorta; LADCA: left anterior descending coronary artery; LCxCA: left circumflex coronary artery; LMCA: left main coronary artery.

F. 5.16. Coronal plane obtained by a fat-supressed rapid breath-hold sequence, especially designed for the study of the coronary vessels, where it is possible to observe the origin and the course of the first portion of the right coronary artery (arrow). AAo: ascending aorta; LV: left ventricle; MPA: main pulmonary artery; RCA: right coronary artery; RV: right ventricle.

F. 5.17. Coronal plane contiguous to that of Figure 5.16, showing a larger extent of the course of the right coronary artery (arrow). LV: left ventricle; RCA: right coronary artery; RV: right ventricle.

F. 5.18. Origin and initial course, crossing anteriorly to the pulmonary trunk, of a saphenous coronary artery bypass graft to the left anterior descending artery (arrows). Images obtained in spin echo T1 (A) and gradient echo techniques (B) are shown. AAo: ascending aorta; BGLAD: bypass graft to the left anterior descending artery; MPA: main pulmonary artery.

F. 5.19. Image of a patent venous bypass graft to the left coronary artery system (in this case to the left circumflex) seen as a circular flow signal anterior to the main pulmonary artery (arrow) in this spin echo sagittal plane. AAo: ascending aorta; AoA: aortic arch; BGCx: bypass graft to the circumflex; LA: left atrium; MPA: main pulmonary artery; RA: right atrium; RV: right ventricle.

FIGURE 5.20 A and B

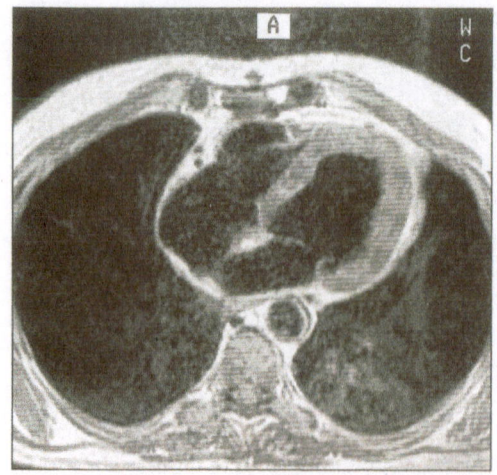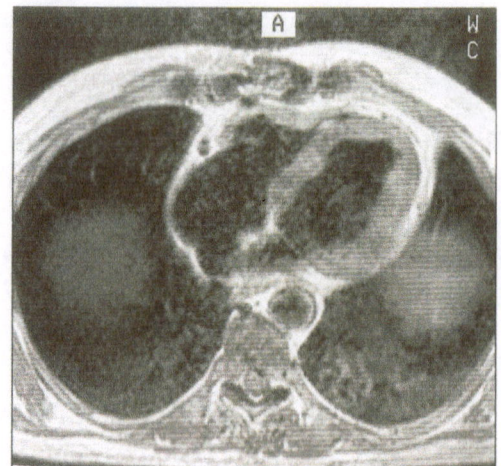

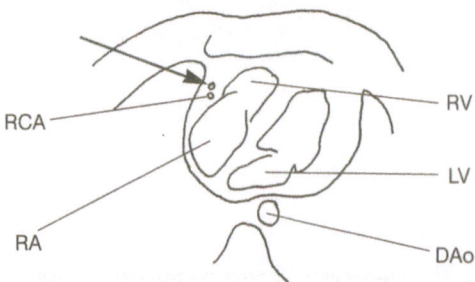

RCA

RV

LV

RA

DAo

FIGURE 5.21 A and B

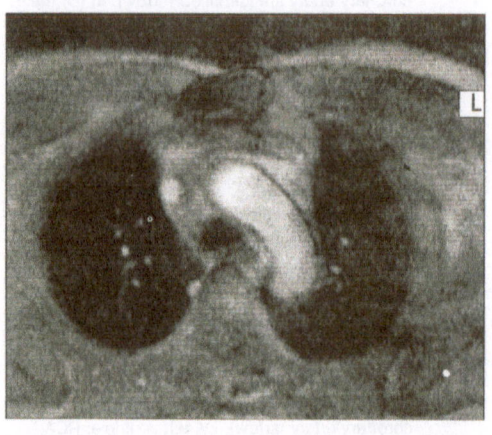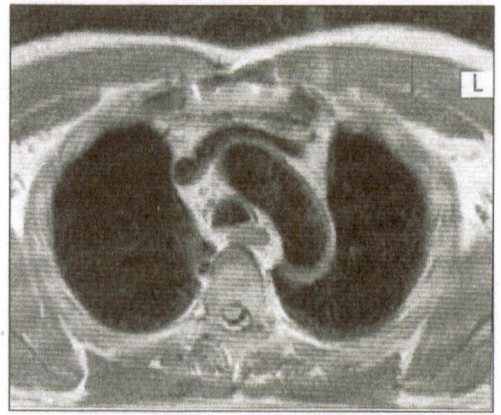

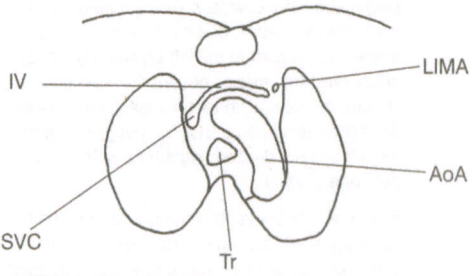

IV

LIMA

AoA

SVC

Tr

This would be complemented, in the near future, with the possibility of imaging the coronary arteries and of measuring the velocity of coronary blood flow and, also, with the evaluation of cardiac energetic metabolism by MRI spectroscopy[36,37]. Improvements in magnetic resonance hardware, software and imaging speed will permit the performance of all of these methods in a simultaneous integrated examination[38,39] (Table 5.1).

Table 5.1 Integrated 'one-stop shop' study of ischemic heart disease using MRI

- Cardiovascular anatomical morphology (size of cavities, thickness of ventricular walls, ventricular mass, post-AMI remodeling, thrombus)
- Global and regional ventricular contractility
- Myocardial perfusion studies with paramagnetic contrasts, at rest and under pharmalogical stress
- Morphological assessment of the coronary tree and assessment of coronary artery bypass graft patency and function
- Myocardial metabolism study by MR spectroscopy

References

1. Budinger TF, Berson A, Mc Veigh ER, et al. Cardiac MR imaging : report of a working group sponsored by the National Heart, Lung, and Blood Institute. Radiology 1998; 208: 573–6.

2. Van der Wall EE, Vliegen HW, de Roos A, Bruschke AVG. Magnetic resonance imaging in coronary artery disease. Circulation 1995; 92: 2723–39.

3. Johnston DL. Myocardial tissue characterization with magnetic resonance imaging techniques. Am J Cardiac Imaging 1994; 8: 140–50.

4. Uokawa K, Nakano Y, Urayama S, et al. An improved computer method to prepare 3D magnetic resonance images of thoracic structures. J Digit Imaging 1997; 10: 85–95.

5. van der Wall EE, van Rugge FP, Vliegen HW, Reiber JH, de Roos A, Bruschke AV. Ischemic heart disease: value of MR techniques. Int J Cardiac Imaging 1997; 13: 179–80.

6. Bexerman JL, Mosher TJ, McVeigh ER, Atalar E, Lima JA, Bluemke DA. Advanced MR techniques for evaluation of the heart and great vessels. Radiographics 1998; 18: 543–64.

7. Baer FM, Theissen P, Voth E, Schneider CA, Schicha H, Sechtem U. Morphologic correlate of pathologic Q waves as assessed by gradient-echo magnetic resonance imaging. Am J Cardiol 1994; 74: 430–4.

8. de Roos A, Niezen RA, Lamb HJ, Dendale P, Reiber JH, van der Wall EE. MR of the heart under pharmacologic stress. Cardiol Clin 1998; 16: 247–65.

9. Matheijssen NAA, Baur LHB, Reiber JHC, et al. Assessment of left ventricular volume and mass by cine magnetic resonance imaging in patients with anterior myocardial infarction intra-observer and inter-observer variability on contour detection. Int J Cardiac Imaging 1996; 12: 11–9.

10. Foster RE, Johnson DB, Barilla F, et al. Changes in left ventricular mass and volumes in patients receiving angiotensin-converting enzyme inhibitor therapy for left ventricular dysfunction after Q-wave myocardial infarction. Am Heart J 1998; 136: 269–75.

11. García-Dorado D, Oliveras J, Gili J, et al. Analysis of myocardial oedema by magnetic resonance imaging early after coronary artery occlusion with or without reperfusion. Cardiovasc Res 1993; 27: 1462–9.

12. Vliegen HW, de Roos A, Brushke AVG, Van del Wall EE. Magnetic resonance techniques for the assessment of myocardial viability: clinical experience. Am Heart J 1995; 129: 809–18.

13. Geschwind JF, Saeed M, Wendland MF, Higgins CB. Depiction of reperfused myocardial infarction using contrast-enhanced spin echo and gradient echo magnetic resonance imaging. Invest Radiol 1998; 33: 386–92.

F. 5.20. Contiguous spin echo axial planes (A: cranial; and B: caudal) in a patient with a saphenous vein bypass graft to the right coronary artery: the relations between the bypass vessel (arrow) and the native right coronary artery are seen. DAo: descending aorta; LA: left atrium; LV: left ventricle; RA: right atrium; RCA: right coronary artery; RV: right ventricle.

F. 5.21. Gradient echo (A) and spin echo (B) images showing the signal elicited by a patent left internal mammary artery graft (arrows): the presence of blood flow in the vessel is depicted as a bright dot in the gradient echo sequence and as a dark signal in the spin echo sequence. AoA: aortic arch; IV: innominate vein; LIMA: left internal mammary artery graft; SVC: superior vena cava.

14. Kramer CM, Rogers WJ, Geskin G, et al. Usefulness of magnetic resonance imaging early after acute myocardial infarction. Am J Cardiol 1997; 15: 690–5.

15. Jungehhlsing M, Sechtem U, Theissen P, Hilger HH, Schicha H. Left ventricular thrombi: evaluation with spin-echo and gradient-echo MR imaging. Radiology 1992; 182: 225–9.

16. Martin ET, Fuisz AR, Pohost GM. Imaging cardiac structure and function. Cardiol Clin 1998; 16: 135–60.

17. Axel L. Noninvasive measurement of cardiac strain with MRI. Adv Exp Med Biol 1997; 430: 249–56.

18. Pattynama PMT, Lamb HJ, Van der Velde EA, Van der Wall EE, de Roos A. Left ventricular measurements with cine and spin-echo MR imaging: a study of reproducibility with variance component analysis. Radiology 1993; 187: 261–8.

19. Pattynama PMT, Lamb HJ, Van der Velde EA, Van der Geest R, Van der Wall EE, de Roos A. Reproducibility of MRI-derived measurements of right ventricular volumes and myocardial mass. Magn Reson Imaging 1995; 13: 77–89.

20. Nachtomy E, Cooperstein R, Vaturi M, Bosak E, Vered Z, Akselrod S. Automatic assessment of cardiac function from short-axis MRI: procedure and clinical evaluation. Magn Reson Imaging 1998; 16: 365–76.

21. McVeigh ER. MRI of myocardial function: motion tracking techniques. Magn Reson Imaging 1996; 14: 137–50.

22. van Rugge FP, van der Wall EE, Spanjersberg SJ, et al. Magnetic resonance imaging during dobutamine stress for detection and localization of coronary artery disease. Circulation 1994; 90: 127–38.

23. Upton MT, Rerych SK, Newman GE, Port S, Cobb FR, Jones RH. Detecting abnormalities in left ventricular function during exercise before angina and ST-segment depression. Circulation 1980; 62: 341–9.

24. Baer FM, Smolarz K, Jungehulsing M, et al. Feasibility of high-dose dipyridamole-magnetic resonance imaging for the detection of coronary artery disease and comparison with coronary angiography. Am J Cardiol 1992; 70: 34–40.

25. Baer FM, Voth E, Theissen P, Schicha H, Sechtem U. Gradient-echo magnetic resonance imaging during incremental dobutamine infusion for the localization of coronary artery stenoses. Eur Heart J 1994; 15: 218–25.

26. Baer F, Voth E, Schneider CA, Theissen P, Schicha H, Sechtem U. Comparison of low-dose dobutamine-gradient-echo magnetic resonance imaging and positron emission tomography with {[18]F} fluorodeoxyglucose in patients with chronic coronary artery disease. Circulation 1995; 91: 1006–15.

27. Manning WJ, Li W, Edelman RR. A preliminary report comparing magnetic resonance coronary angiography with conventional angiography. N Engl J Med 1993; 328: 828–32.

28. Pennell DJ, Keegan J, Firmin DN, Gatehouse PD, Underwood SR, Longmore DB. Magnetic resonance imaging of coronary arteries: technique and preliminary results. Br Heart J 1993; 70: 315–26.

29. Pons-Lladó G. Estado actual del estudio de las arterias coronarias y los injertos quirúrgicos por métodos no invasivos. Rev Esp Cardiol 1998; 51: 510–20.

30. Post JC, van Rossum AC, Hofman MB, Valk J, Visser CA. Three-dimensional respiratory-gated MR angiography of coronary arteries: comparison with conventional coronary angiography. Am J Roentgenol 1996; 166: 1399–404.

31. Dinsmore RE. Noninvasive coronariography. Here at last? Circulation 1995; 91: 1607–8.

32. Hundley WG, Clarke GD, Landau Ch, et al. Noninvasive determination of infarct artery patency by cine magnetic resonance angiography. Circulation 1995; 91 :1347–53.

33. Di Renzi P, Fedele F, Di Cesare E, et al. Identification of coronary artery by-pass grafts: reliability of MRI in clinical practice. Int J Card Imaging 1992; 8: 85–94.

34. Furber A, Sakuma H, Higgins CB. Contribution of MRI in the evaluation of ischemic heart diseases. Arch Mal Coeur Vaiss 1997; 90: 1501–10.

35. Pons Lladó G, Carreras F. Estado actual de las aplicaciones de la resonancia magnética en el estudio de la cardiopatía isquémica. Rev Esp Cardiol 1997; 50: 59–73.

36. Yabe T, Mitsunami K, Inubushi T, Kinoshita M. Quantitative measurements of cardiac phosphorus metabolites in coronary artery disease by 31P magnetic resonance spectroscopy. Circulation 1995; 92: 15–23.

37. Neubaer S, Horn M, Hahn D, Kochsiek K. Clinical cardiac magnetic resonance spectroscopy. Present state and future directions. Mol Cell Biochem 1998; 184: 439–43.

38. Kramer CM. Integrated approach to ischemic heart disease. The one-stop shop. Cardiol Clin 1998; 16: 267–76.

39. Blackwell GG, Pohost GM. The evolving role of MRI in the assessment of coronary artery disease. Am J Cardiol 1995; 75: 74D–78D.

Cardiac and paracardiac masses

6

F. CARRERAS-COSTA

6.1 Introduction

Cardiac tumors are a rare cause of heart disease, being found in autopsy series with a frequency ranging between 0.0017% and 0.03%[1], 30% are myxomas and 20–30% are malignancies, almost always sarcomas. Cardiac metastases are 10 to 40 times more frequent than primary heart cancer. The diagnosis of the presence of a tumor involving the cardiovascular system in live patients was difficult in the past due to the elusive character of clinical signs and symptoms, their recognition being usually made at post-mortem examinations (Table 6.1)[2]. Radiology and angiography were the first techniques that permitted the diagnosis, although restricted to those masses that were of sufficient size to cause radiological or hemodynamic manifestations. The introduction of echocardiography radically changed the diagnostic process, particularly with the availability of transesophageal techniques[3]. Cardiac tumors or masses are frequently an unsuspected finding in asymptomatic patients, their clinical manifestations, when present, being related to their localization, size or behavior, causing pericardial effusion (metastases, mesotheliomas), compression of the cavities (cysts, thymomas, lymphomas), myocardial restriction (fibromas, hemangiomas, sarcomas), paroxysmal pulmonary congestion (myxomas), or peripheral embolism (thrombi, papillary fibroelastoma). Although a first line diagnostic tool, echocardiography does have limitations: poor image quality in those cases with a difficult acoustic window, and limited field of vision, especially for paracardiac masses[4,5,6]. In the latter, the differential diagnosis is frequently challenging as extrinsic cardiac compression may be due to many different causes such as pleural effusion, hiatus hernia, or, simply, a chest wall malformation as in pectus excavatum[7].

MRI is the most recent imaging technique added to the diagnostic armamentarium[8]. The importance of the information obtained from its images has raised MRI to an important position in the field of diagnostic techniques, complementing or even surpassing echocardiography on many occasions[9]. It is preferred to computerized tomography (CT) because of its superior image resolution and the possibility of obtaining angulated image planes, although the detection of calcifications remains one of the few advantages of CT (Table 6.2). It should be kept in mind, however, that false-positive diagnoses can occur, especially when dealing with atrial fibromuscular structures, that can look like masses (thrombi)[10]. Experience is, therefore, necessary in the evaluation of MRI studies in order to increase the diagnostic specificity of the technique and avoid pitfalls from the misinterpretation of normal structures.

6.2 Technical Aspects in the Evaluation of Masses with MRI

The excellent soft tissue MRI definition permits the sharp delineation of the myocardium, pericardium, paracardiac fat, vascular structures and the lungs, and thus facilitates the identification and study of abnormal masses. The wide field of vision permits unlimited observation of the extension and the anatomical relationships of cardiac and paracardiac masses with the great

Table 6.1   Classification of the most frequent primary and secondary cardiac tumors

Primary		Secondary		
Benign	Malignant	Direct extension	Venous extension	Metastatic extension
Myxoma	Sarcoma	Lung carcinoma	Renal cell carcinoma	Melanoma
Pericardial cyst	Mesothelioma	Breast carcinoma	Adrenal carcinoma	Leukemia
Lipoma	Lymphoma	Esophageal carcinoma	Hepatocellular carcinoma	Lymphoma
Fibroelastoma	Other	Mediastinal tumors	Thyroid carcinoma	Genitourinary tract
Rhabdomyoma			Carcinoma of the lung	Gastronitestinal tract
Fibroma			Sarcoma of the uterus	
Hemangioma				

Table 6.2   Usefulness of different diagnostic techniques for the study of cardiac tumors*

	x-ray	Computerized tomography	Angiography	Echocardiography	MRI
Primary benign					
Myxoma	+	++	+++	+++++	++++
Pericardial cyst	++	+++	0	+	+++++
Lipoma	+	+++	+	+++	+++++
Fibroelastoma	0	0	0	+++++	+++
Rhabdomyoma	0	+	+	+++++	++++
Fibroma	0	+	+	++++	++++
Primary malignant					
Sarcoma	+	++	++	+++	+++++
Mesothelioma	+	+++	+	++	+++++
Lymphoma	++	+++	+	++	+++++
Secondary tumors					
Direct proliferation	+	+++	++	+++	+++++
Venous proliferation	0	+	+++	++++	++++
Metastases	+	++	+	++	++++

0: not useful; +: limited use; ++: may be used; +++: useful; ++++: very useful; +++++: preferred diagnostic test. * Taken from Salcedo EE, et al.

vessels and the bronchial tree, information that is especially useful to guide surgeons in the design of an appropriate therapeutic strategy[11,12].

To some extent, MRI allows some degree of tumor tissue characterization[13], in particular of those tumors with a high fat content, such as lipomas, which stand out for their bright signal intensity in T1 spin echo sequences (Figure 6.1).

A comparative analysis of signal intensity characteristics by the different sequences available in MRI allows a quite reliable evaluation of the composition of the mass under study (Table 6.3). Comparing the characteristics of the same image in T1 and T2 spin echo sequences (Figure 6.2), the composition of an effusion or cyst can be assessed, although it should be noted that the signal of the hematic collections varies according to the degree of hemoglobin decomposition over time (Table 6.4). This information is useful for an approximate dating of the evolution time of a hematoma[14] (Figure 6.3).

An important limitation of T2 spin echo sequences is the poor definition and blurry image that is obtained due to the motion artifacts that are produced by the respiratory movements and the inconstant synchronization with the electrocardiogram imposed by long TR required for these sequences. The presence of hemorrhage or necrosis within the tumor can characteristically alter its appearance (Figure 6.4A). On the other hand, intravenous administration of paramagnetic contrast agents permit imaging of the degree of vascularization, allowing the differentiation between benign and malignant masses (Figure 6.4A), and facilitating the identification of intramyocardial masses[15].

In practice, the decision to use MRI for the evaluation of a cardiac or paracardiac mass is almost always based on a previous echocardiogram in which the existence of a mass was suspected. In our experience, MRI is particularly useful in the study of paracardiac masses, whose clinical manifestations, on many occasions, depend more on the complications due to its anatomical location than on its histological characteristics.

6.3 Malignant Primary Cardiac Tumors

Sarcomas are the most frequent malignancies of this group. They occur mainly in the right atrium and, as a result, may occlude inflow into the atrium from either vena cava, as well as obstruct right ventricular outflow. The tumors are named for the dominant cellular element involved.

a. Angiosarcoma

Angiosarcomas are one of the most common tumors we can encounter in this group. Figure 6.4A shows a patient affected by an angiosarcoma of a pericardial origin appearing as an intramural mass of the right atrial wall, where such tumors are usually found[16]. The patient underwent surgery, the tumor was resected and the right atrial wall was reconstructed using a pericardium patch (Figure 6.4B). The clinical follow-up was in accordance with other cases described in the literature; the patient died a few months following surgery due to disseminated metastases[17,18].

b. Myxosarcoma

The diagnosis of atrial myxosarcoma is difficult for the pathologist and sometimes can be erroneously diagnosed as a myxoma[19]. This case happened to a young patient in which an intraventricular mass was diagnosed by echocardiography. A thorough preoperative investigation was accomplished by MRI (Figure 6.5A), and no evidence of metastatic lesions was established jointly with other techniques. A preoperative direct biopsy of the tumor was not conclusive for malignancy, suggesting a diagnosis of myxoma, and the mass was surgically fully resected. Because of the involvement of mitral valve apparatus, the mitral valve was resected and a metallic prosthesis implanted. Unfortunately, a more exhaustive pathological examination was carried out and the diagnosis of myxosarcoma was definitely confirmed. The tumor relapsed in a few months (Figure 6.5B).

FIGURE 6.1A and B

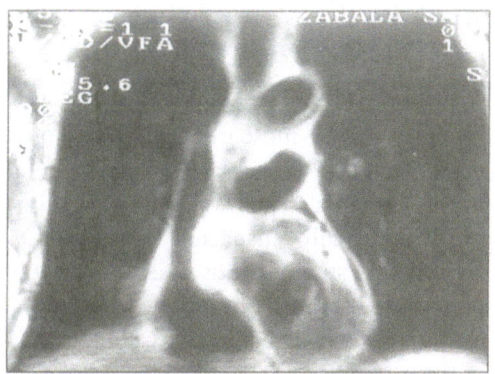
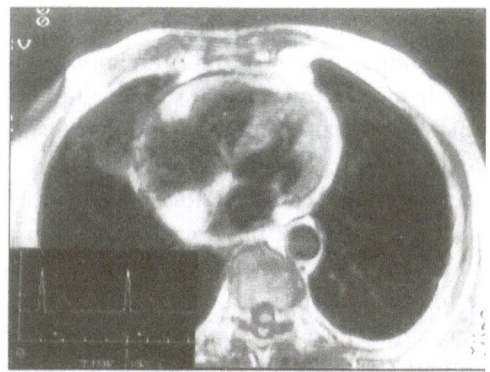

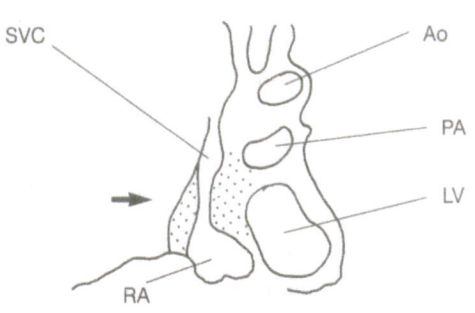
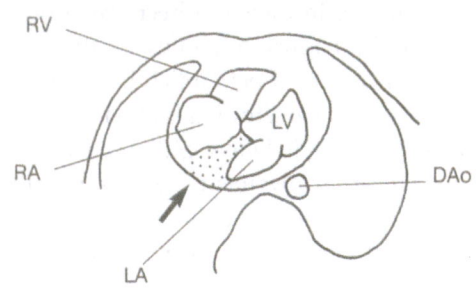

FIGURE 6.2A and B

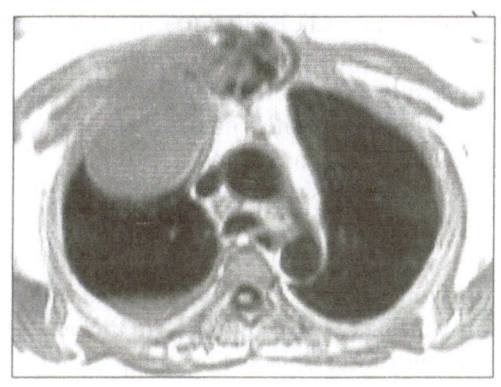
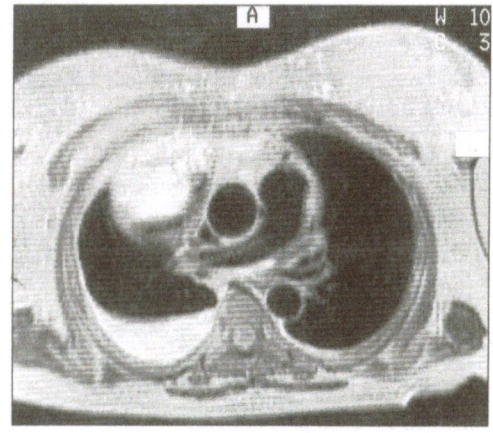

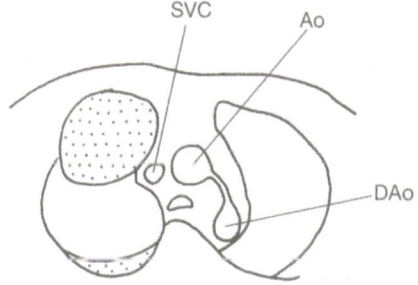
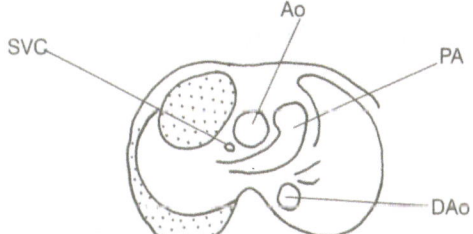

F. 6.1. Characteristic hyperintense signal (white) of a lipoma obtained in T1 weighted spin echo. In the sagittal plane (A) the tumor is seen surrounding the superior vena cava (arrow). In an axial slice (B) the involvement of the superior segment of the interatrial septal wall is observed (arrow). Ao: aorta; DAo: descending aorta; LA: left atrium; LV: left ventricle; PA: pulmonary artery; RA: right atrium; RV: right ventricle; SVC: superior vena cava.

F. 6.2. Late subacute postoperative mediastinal hematoma and right hemothorax (dotted areas) studied in spin-echo T1 (A) and T2 (B) sequences. The T2 sequence depicts a characteristically bright signal from both hematic collections (see table 6.4). Ao: aorta; DAo: descending aorta; PA: pulmonary artery: SVC: superior vena cava.

84

c. Pericardial tumors

Secondary metastatic infiltration of the pericardium (breast and lung carcinomas, melanomas, leukemia and lymphoma)[20] is much more frequent than primary tumors (mesothelioma). Primary tumors can manifest themselves as a mass in the pericardial sac; therefore, a differential diagnosis in order to avoid confusing fibrin aggregates with a tumor should be considered in those patients with chronic pericardial effusion (Figure 6.6). Pericardial involvement due to secondary tumors occurs by direct extension or via the bloodstream. In cases of direct extension, a loss of the normal continuity of the pericardium, abnormal pericardial thickening or the presence of an effusion is observed using MRI (Figure 6.7). In hematogenous dissemination, focal involvement due to nodular lesions, enlargement or also effusion, nearly always hemorrhagic, is usually observed.

Table 6.3 Differential diagnosis of an image of cardiac mass according to MR signal intensity (SI) characteristics

High SI on spin echo T1:
   fat, effect of paramagnetic contrast, recent subacute hemorrhage (1 to 3 days)
Intermediate SI on T1 and high on T2:
   tumor, thrombus, cyst with elevated protein content
Low SI in T1 and very high on T2:
   serous cyst
Intermediate SI on gradient echo:
   tumor
Low SI on gradient echo:
   thrombus

6.4 Benign Primary Cardiac Tumors

a. Lipomas

Lipomas are the most frequently diagnosed benign tumors[21]. They are generally found in the interatrial septal wall, and their diagnosis is usually suspected based on an echographic study. In this case, MRI is the preferred diagnostic technique due to its ability to clearly detect the fatty composition of the tumor (Figure 6.1).

b. Pericardial masses and tumors

The most frequent benign disorders are pericardial cysts[20] (see chapter 7), which, depending on their location, can cause hemodynamic compromise. Cysts should show a low intensity signal in spin echo T1 and high signal intensity in T2, although if they contain a high amount of fibrin or are hematic, the T1 signal can be of an intermediate or high signal intensity.

An exceptional case in our series is that of a patient who presented with an intrapericardial mass of relatively homogeneous characteristics, with intermediate signal intensity on T1, increasing heterogeneously on T2 (Figure 6.6A and B), and compressing the right ventricle (Figure 6.6C). The mass was surgically removed and turned out to be a large fibrin aggregate in the pericardial cavity. The "malignancy" stemmed from the hemodynamic consequences of the compression of the right cavities.

c. Myocardial tumors

The differential diagnosis of malignant tumors is usually difficult, since there are no specific

Table 6.4 Evolution of signal intensity (SI) of a hemorrhage related to time

Condition	Time	Hemoglobin	T1 SI	T2 SI
Acute	< 24 hours	Oxyhemoglobin	Intermediate	Intermediate
Recent subacute	1–3 days	Deoxyhemoglobin	High*	Intermediate
Late subacute	3–14 days	Metahemoglobin	Intermediate**	High
Chronic	> 14 days	Hemosiderin***	Low	Low

* Homogeneous signal
** Heterogeneous signal (intermediate/high)
*** The accumulation of hemosiderin produces a very low or even absent SI. The null image of the liver parenchyma is very characteristic in hemochromatosis or secondary hemosiderosis, as in patients that have received numerous blood transfusions or hemodialysis (Figure 6.3B)

FIGURE 6.3A and B

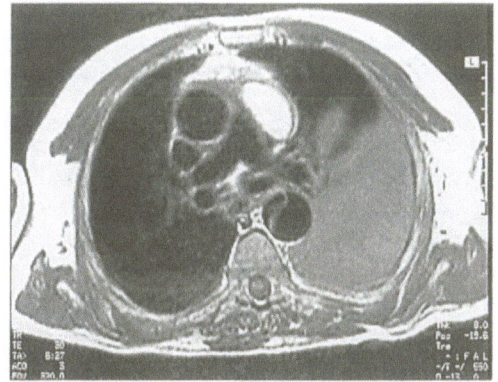

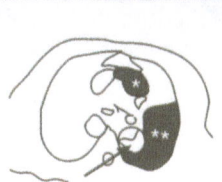

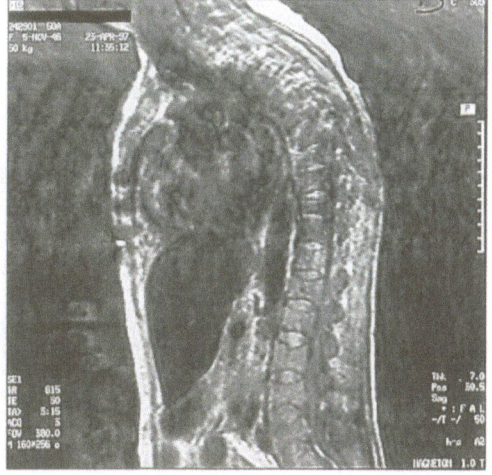

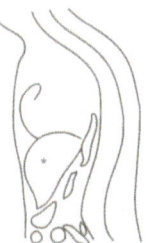

FIGURE 6.4A and B

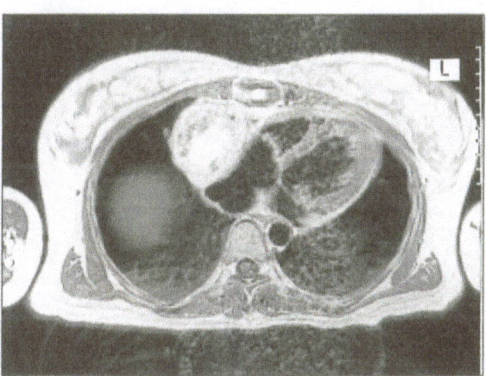

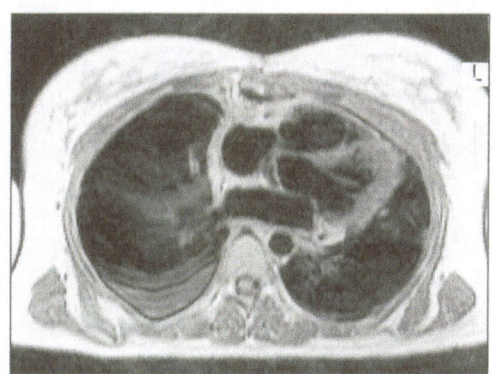

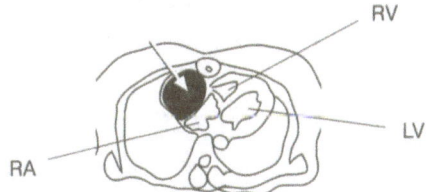

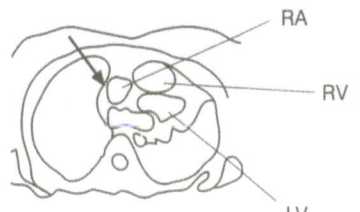

F. 6.3.   (A) T1 weighted spin echo image of a patient with a type B aortic dissection (arrow) obtained 36 hours after the first clinical symptoms. A para-aortic hematoma that extends to the ascending aorta (*) and a significant hemothorax (**) can be observed. The hemorrhage signal is hyperintense in the para-aortic area, corresponding to a recent subacute hemorrhage, and intermediate in the hemothorax, which in turn corresponds to an acute hemorrhage that should have occurred after the para-aortic one. (B) Sagittal T1 weighted spin echo image of a patient affected by hepatic hemosiderosis; no MRI signal can be observed in the hepatic parenchyma.

F. 6.4.   (A) T1 weighted spin echo image of a hemangiosarcoma affecting the right atrium (arrow) following the administration of gadolinium-DTPA. A marked increase in the intensity of the tumor due to contrast uptake is observed. The hyperintense signal (white) in the interior corresponds to an area of subacute hemorrhage. (B) Image obtained following resection of the hemangiosarcoma, the right atrial wall having been reconstructed by means of a pericardial patch (arrow). RA: right atrium; LA: left atrium; RV: right ventricle; LV: left ventricle

FIGURE 6.5A

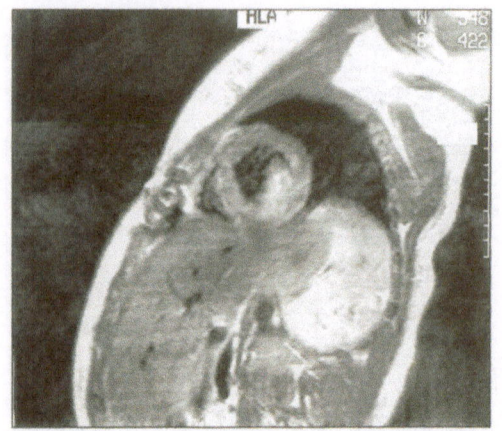

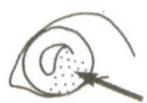

FIGURE 6.6A,B,C

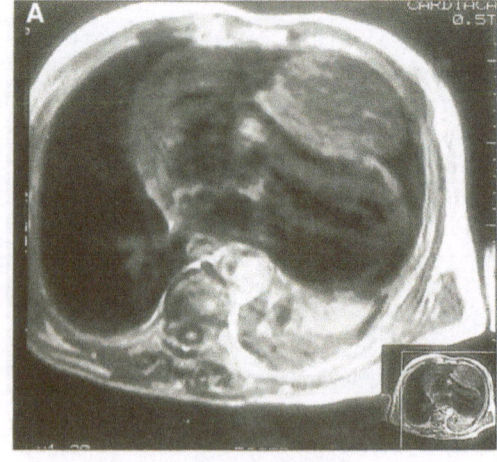

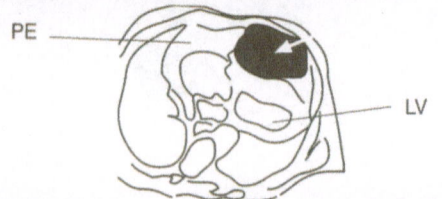

FIGURE 6.5B

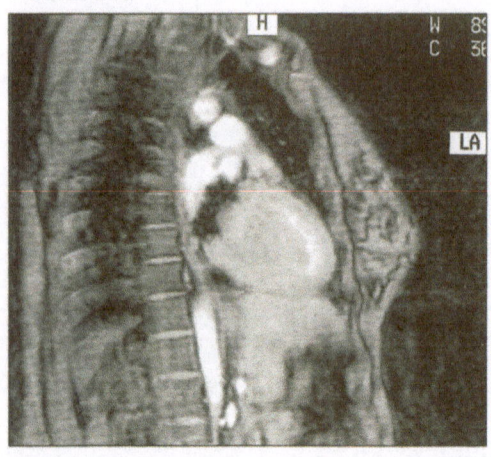

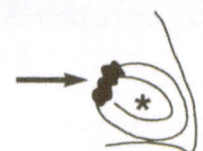

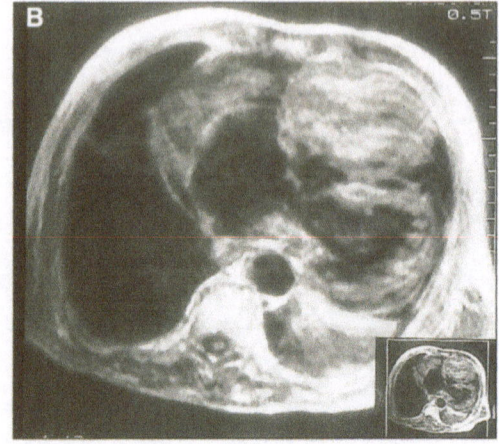

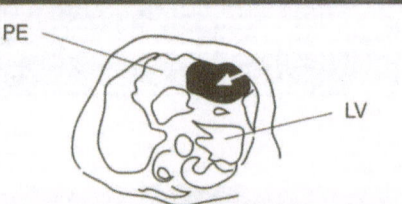

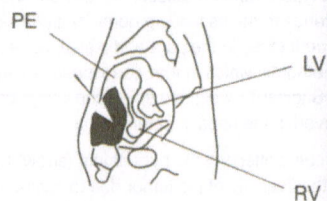

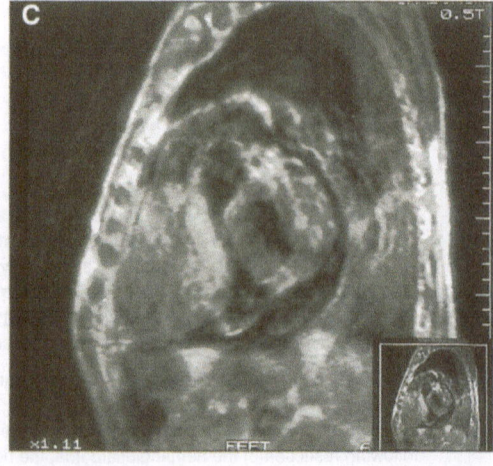

differential characteristics. Nevertheless, benign tumors, due to the fact that they grow slowly, are usually of a relatively homogeneous signal intensity, although in the case of the hemangiomas this is not the rule due to their vascular composition (Figure 6.8). Malignant tumors, which grow rapidly, normally contain foci of hemorrhage or necrosis.

Benign primary intramyocardial tumors, such as hemangiomas[22], fibromas[23] (Figure 6.9A and B) or rhabdomyomas, the latter being more frequent in infancy, must be distinguished from hypertrophic cardiomyopathy with marked segmental involvement (Figure 6.9C). In order to accomplish this, it is helpful to use T2 spin echo sequences or administer contrast agents: the tumors will stand out due to the marked increase in their signal intensity.

6.5   Secondary Cardiac Tumors

a. Mediastinal lymphomas

Malignant hematological processes involving the mediastinum are the most frequent cases of this group, lymphomas in particular[24], which give rise to a mass of homogeneous characteristics of intermediate density that increase with the administration of gadolinium. Mediastinal infiltration is usually extensive, frequently involving the vascular structures, either by infiltration or by compression. Cardiovascular involvement can be manifested in various ways. When the superior mediastinum is predominantly involved, superior vena cava compression is frequent, leading to a characteristic type of edema which manifests intself in a collar-shaped fashion in the superior half of the chest (Figure 6.10). If the infiltration involves the posterior mediastinum, compression of the left atrium and the pulmonary veins is

observed. On occasions, the involvement is localized in the anterior mediastium, and cardiac structures such as the right atrium are selectively compressed, and even the pericardium can be infiltrated (Figure 6.7). Retroperitoneal fibrosis with mediastinal involvement is a rare condition that must be distinguished from lymphomas. Figure 6.11 presents a patient affected with this condition. The fibrotic mass surrounds the abdominal aorta and its branches (Figure 6.11A), and spreads to the mediastinum traversing the diaphragm. The progression of the mass surrounds intramediastinal large vessels and the heart, infiltrating the right atrial wall and the anterior parietal pericardium (Figure 6.11B).

b. Lung neoplasms

Lung carcinomas can also cause compression (Figure 6.12) or infiltration either of the pericardium (Figure 6.13) or of the cardiac structures by direct extension via the pulmonary veins (Figure 6.14).

6.6   Benign Paracardiac Masses or Pseudotumors

Although the majority are first detected by echocardiography, frequently it is not possible to establish a precise diagnosis. MRI is therefore indicated. These are some examples from our experience:

- Masses of a vascular origin, such as an aortic pseudoaneurysm of mycotic origin, located in the root of the vessel (Figure 6.15A), which was diagnosed by transesophageal echocardiography but appropriately delimited by MRI. This information was useful to the surgeon, who decided not to resect but to seal its

F. 6.5.   Transverse left ventricular spin echo T1 sequence depicting the presence of a intraventricular myocardial mass, enhanced after gadolinium-DTPA administration (arrow) (A). After a complete surgical resection a diagnosis of myxosarcoma was made. The mass relapsed a few months later, occupying the left ventricular cavity again (asterisk), as shown in a gradient echo sequence (B). Note the artifact of the metallic mitral valve prosthesis (arrow).

F. 6.6.   Pericardial pseudotumor that corresponds to a fibrin mass (arrow) with defined edges and a homogeneous intensity in T1 weighted spin echo sequence (A); the T2 signal is more intense but heterogeneous (B), raising doubts about its true etiology. The unstable hemodynamic situation resulting from its compression of the right ventricle (C) compelled its surgical removal, during which the etiological diagnosis was confirmed. RA: right atrium; PE: pericardial effusion; RV: right ventricle; LV: left ventricle.

FIGURE 6.7A and B

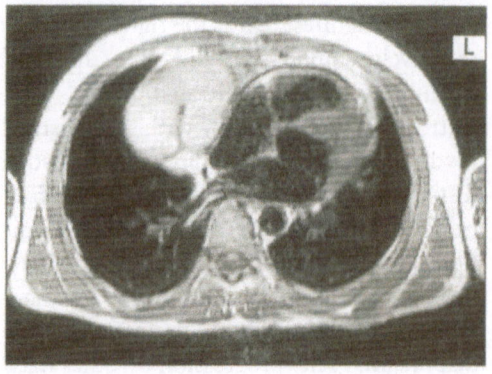
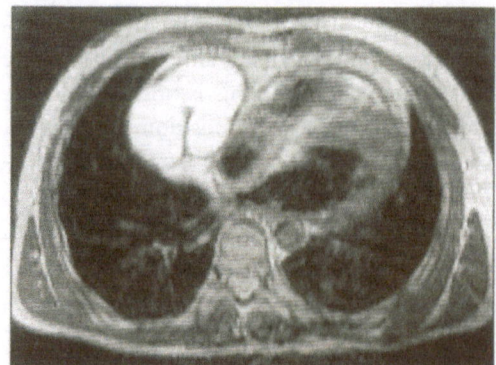

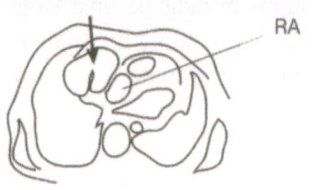
RA

FIGURE 6.8A and B

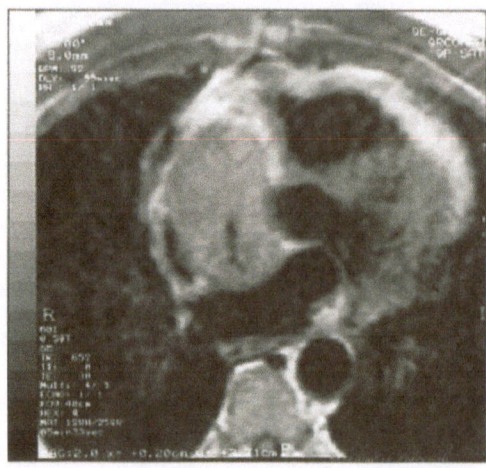
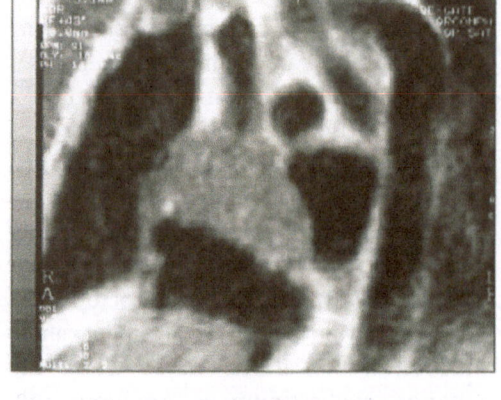

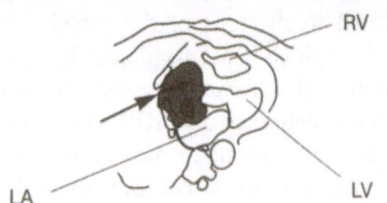
RV
LA
LV

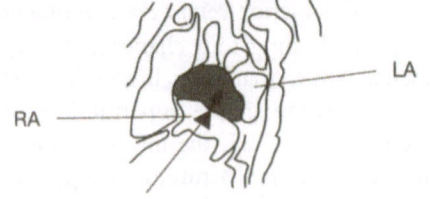
LA
RA

F. 6.7. T1(A) and T2 weighted (B) spin echo image of a right paracardiac lymphoma that infiltrates the pericardium, with loss of continuity of the hypointense line (black) that characterizes it (arrow). Note the increase in signal intensity in the T2 sequence. RA: right atrium.

F. 6.8. T1 weighted spin echo image in axial (A) and sagittal (B) planes of a hemangioma that occupies a large part of the superior half of the right atrium and that displays a slightly heterogeneous intensity due to its vascular structure. RA: right atrium; LA: left atrium; RV: right ventricle; LV: left ventricle.

FIGURE 6.9A

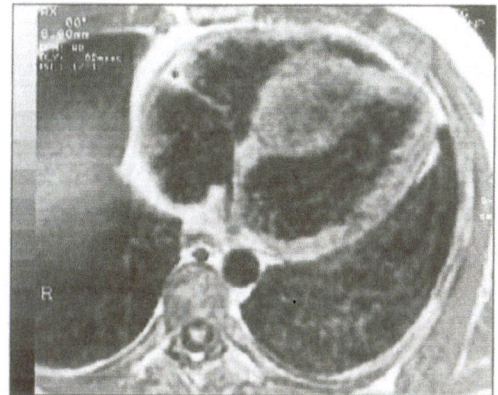

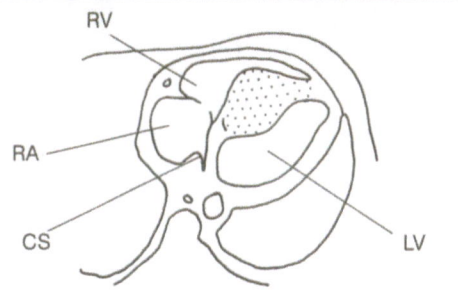

FIGURE 6.9C

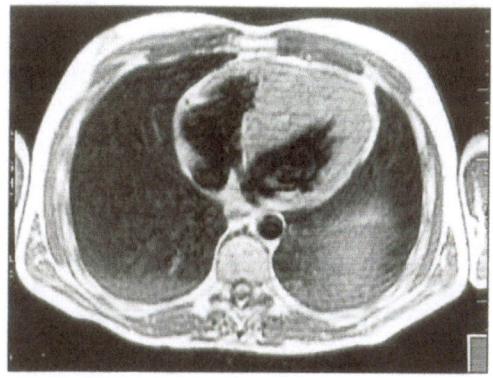

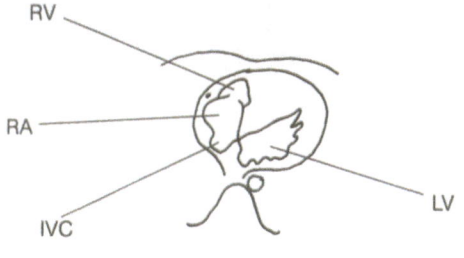

FIGURE 6.9B

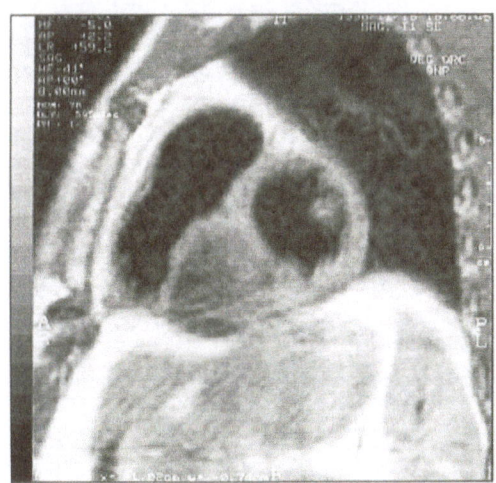

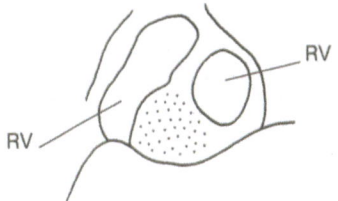

F. 6.9. (A) Axial spin echo plane showing a large increase in thickness of the interventricular septum (dotted area). (B) Sagittal plane in the same case disclosing the presence of a discrete intramural mass involving the interventricular septum at its inferior portion. The mass is indicated by its lower signal intensity than the myocardium (dotted area), which is not infiltrated, as a clear line between the mass and the surrounding myocardial tissue seems to be observed. The mass has the characteristic features of a benign myocardial fibroma. (C) Axial plane in a different patient with severe hypertrophic cardiomyopathy, a condition that should not be misdiagnosed as an intramural tumor, for which the finding of a uniform signal from the hypertrophied myocardium is very useful. CS: coronary sinus; IVC: inferior vena cava; LA: left atrium; LV: left ventricle; RA: right atrium; RV: right ventricle

FIGURE 6.10A and B

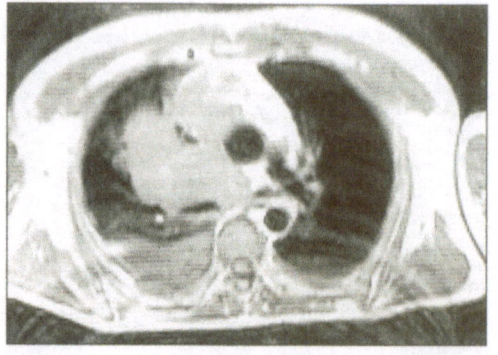
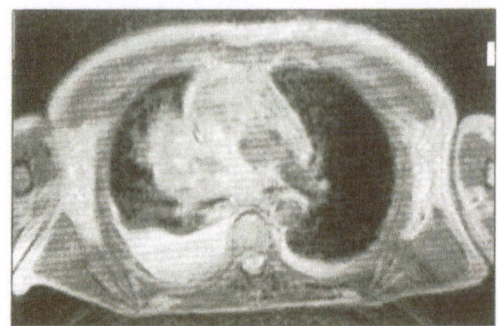

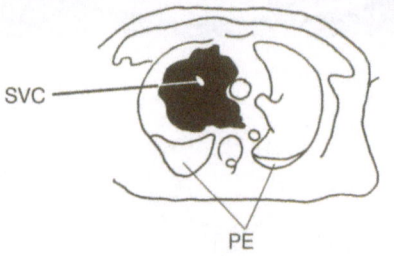

SVC

PE

FIGURE 6.11A and B

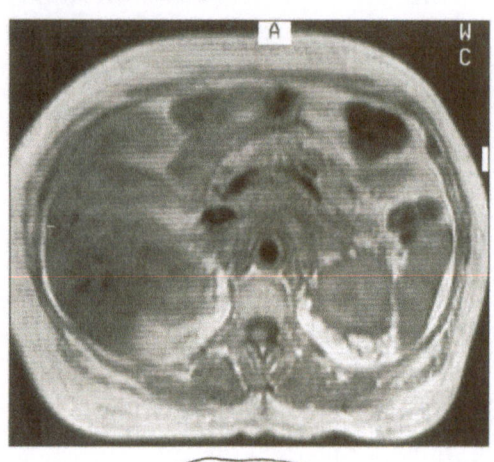
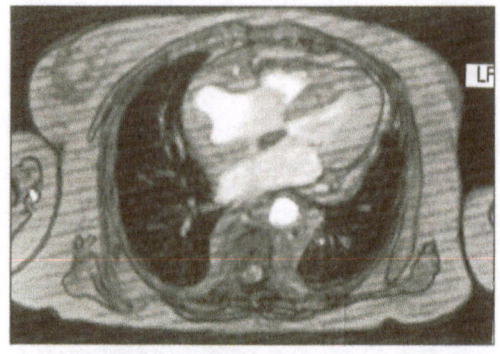

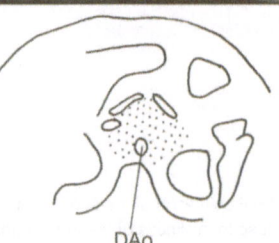

DAo

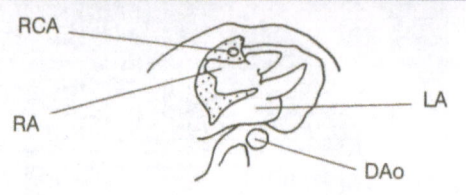

RCA

RA

LA

DAo

PA

SVC

Ao

LA

DAo

FIGURE 6.12

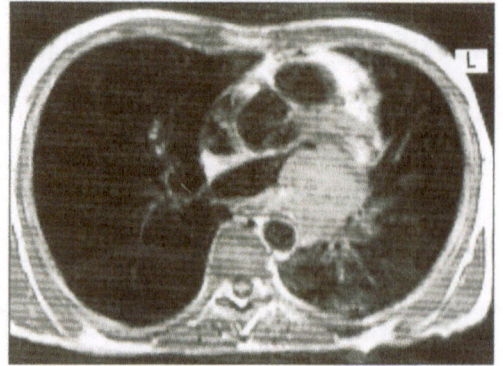

FIGURE 6.13A and B

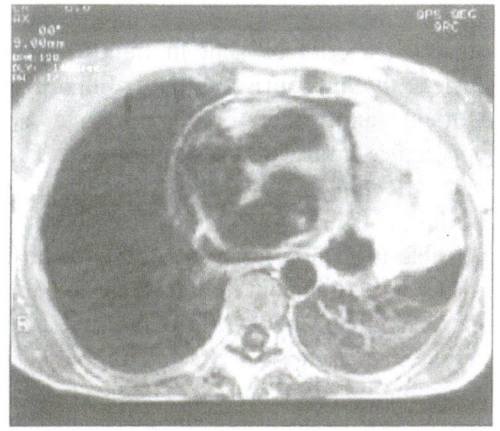

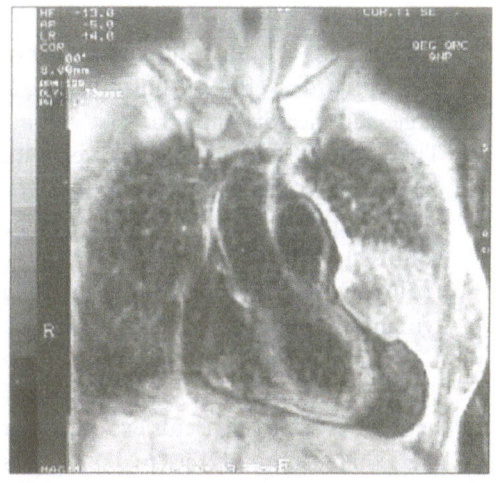

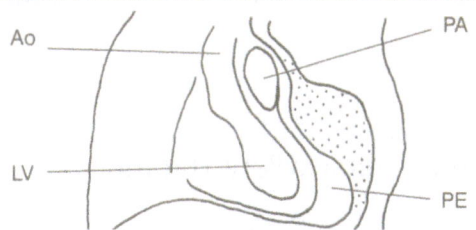

FIGURE 6.14A and B

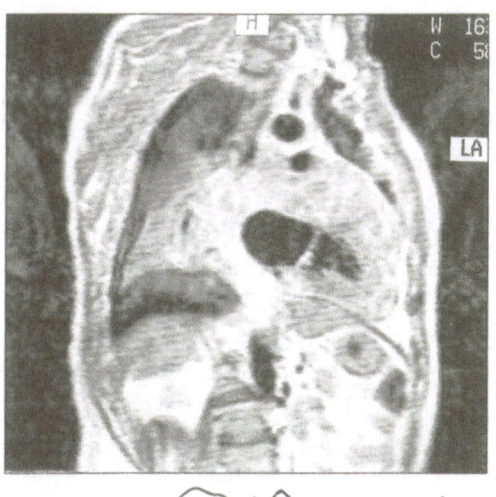

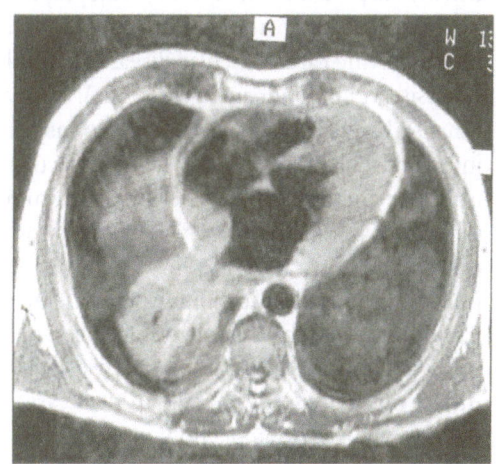

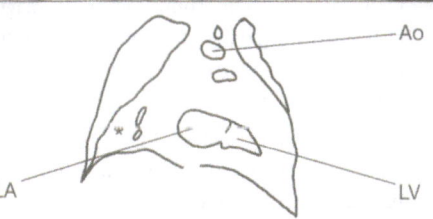

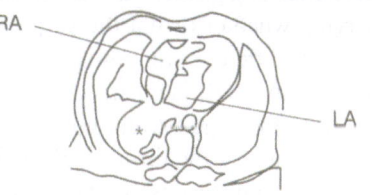

F. 6.10. (A) T1 weighted spin echo image of a mediastinal lymphoma that surrounds and compresses the superior vena cava, practically obstructing its lumen, which greatly hampers its flow. (B) T2 sequence in the same case, showing an increase in signal intensity. Ao: aorta; PA: pulmonary artery; PE: pleural effusion; SVC: superior vena cava.

F. 6.11. T1 spin echo image corresponding to a retroperitoneal fibrosis with mediastinal involvement. The fibrotic mass (dotted area) surrounds the abdominal aorta, that presents a marked increase of its wall thickness, and compresses retroperitoneal structures, in particular the renal vessels and ureters (A). The mediastinal involvement includes infiltration of the right atrial wall and the inter-atrial septum, as shown in a gradient echo sequence (B). Ao: aorta; DAo: descending aorta; LA: left atrium; RA: right atrium; RCA: right coronary artery.

F. 6.12. T1 spin echo image of a bronchial carcinoma compressing the left atrial cavity. Ao: aorta; LA: left atrium; PA: pulmonary artery; SVC: superior vena cava.

F. 6.13. Spin echo axial (A) and coronal (B) images from a patient with primitive lung lymphoma with pericardial infiltration (arrow). Extension of the process to the heart itself is prevented by the pericardium. Note also the presence of pericardial effusion. Ao: aorta; LV: left ventricle; PA: pulmonary artery; PE: pericardial effusion.

F. 6.14. Oblique sagittal (A) and axial (B) spin echo planes in a patient with lung carcinoma (asterisk) infiltrating the myocardium. Ao: aorta; LA: left atrium; LV: left ventricle; RA: right atrium.

connection with the aorta by means of a teflon patch (Figure 6.15B).

- Enlargement of cardiac silhouette due not to a pericardial effusion but rather to a large subepicardial lipoma (Figure 6.16). These disorders are usually detected with echocardiography and, according to the clinical situation of the patient, may be confused with an effusion or an infiltrating mass of the pericardium, such as a lymphoma.

- Deformation and/or compression of the cardiac structures due to a diaphragmatic hernia (Figure 6.17), a pectus excavatum or the combination of the two processes (Figure 6.18).

6.7 Intracavitary Thrombi

The diagnosis of an intracavitary thrombus is usually suspected from an echocardiographic study, according to the clinical context and the coexisting cardiovascular diseases (mitral stenosis, ventricular aneurysm, etc.). They can also be detected by MRI, as is the case of intraventricular thrombi in left ventricular ischemic aneurysms, or intra-atrial thrombi when atrial dilatation or valvular disease exists. Their characteristics in T1 spin echo images are usually indistinguishable from a tumor mass. On the other hand, the presence of blood flow artifacts can be confused with intracavitary masses, especially in those areas of slow blood flow or flow stasis[25]. The differential diagnosis is facilitated by observing whether or not the suspect image persists in different study image planes and by taking cine-MRI gradient echo sequences. Due to its high iron content, it is characteristic that the thrombus signal in the gradient echo images is of a very low intensity (black) (Figure 6.19), standing out against

the high intensity of the flow signal (white), while tumors present with an intermediate signal. It should be kept in mind, nevertheless, that myxomas also have a high iron content and, therefore, can have an appearance similar to that of thrombi[13]. The cine-MR sequence also allows thrombus to be differentiated from the flow artifacts if it is possible to identify the presence of defined mass edges, ruling out flow artifacts. The use of a paramagnetic contrast also aids the differential diagnosis between a tumor and a thrombus.

References

1. McAllister HA. Primary tumors of the heart and pericardium. Curr Probl Cardiol 1979; 4: 1–51.

2. Salcedo EE, Cohen GE, White RD, Davison MB. Cardiac tumors: diagnosis and management. Curr Probl Cardiol 1992; 17(2): 73–137.

3. Mügge A, Daniel WG, Haverich A, Lichtlen PR. Diagnosis of noninfective cardiac mass lesions by two-dimensional echocardiography. Comparison of the transthoracic and transesophageal approaches. Circulation 1991; 83: 70–8.

4. Go RT, O'Donnell JK, Underwood DA, et al. Comparison of gated cardiac MRI and 2D echocardiography of intracardiac neoplasms. Am J Radiol 1985; 145: 21–5.

5. Brown JJ, Barakos JA, Higgins CB. Magnetic resonance imaging of cardiac and paracardiac masses. J Thorac Imag 1989; 4: 58.

6. Freedberg RS, Kronzon I, Rumancik WM, Liebeskind D. The contribution of magnetic resonance imaging to the evaluation of intracardiac tumors diagnosed by echocardiography. Circulation 1988; 77: 96–103.

7. Menegus MA, Greenberg MA, Spindola-Franco H, Fayemi A. Magnetic resonance imaging of suspected atrial tumors. Am Heart J 1992; 123: 1260–8.

F. 6.15. Image from a gradient echo sequence used to study flow circulation in a large mycotic aneurysm (asterisk) arising from the posterior aspect of the artic root, before (A) and after (B) surgical correction. In this latter image there is no active flow inside the aneurysm, as the communication with the aorta had been sealed at surgery. Ao: aorta; LV: left ventricle.

F. 6.16. T1 weighted spin echo angulated sagittal plane depicting a transverse section of the cardiac chambers. A significant accumulation of fat (hyperintense signal) is observed, infiltrating the anterior wall of the right ventricle (dotted area). LV: left ventricle; RV: right ventricle.

FIGURE 6.15A and B

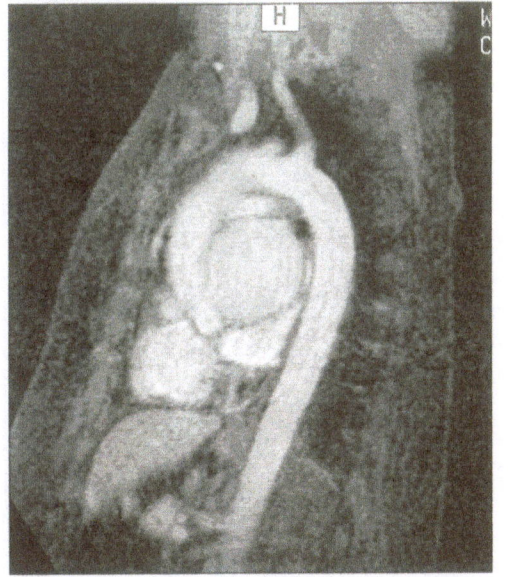

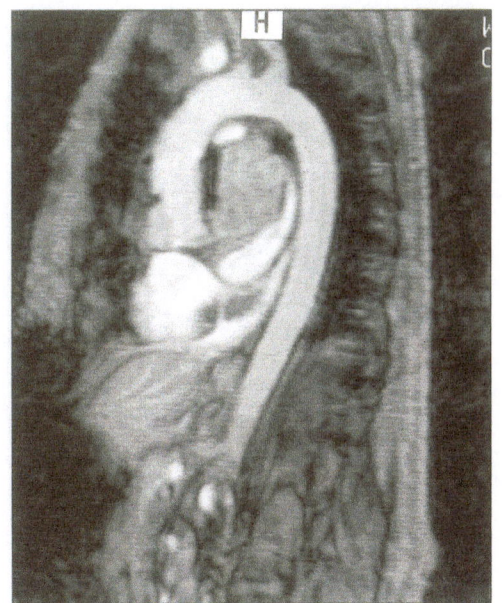

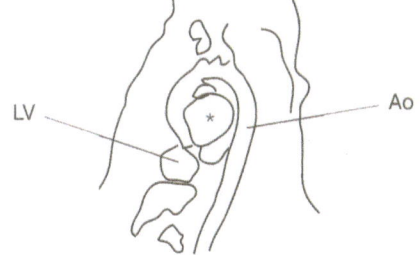

FIGURE 6.16

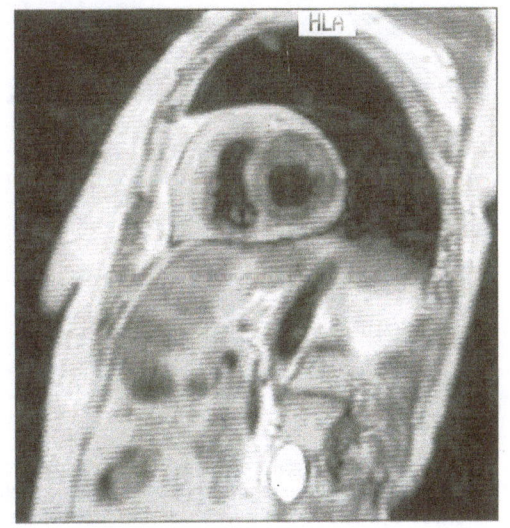

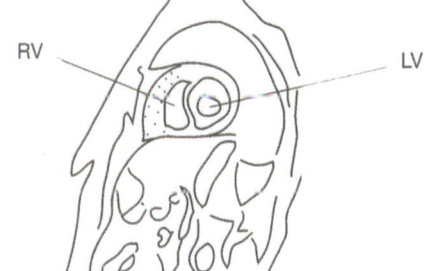

FIGURE 6.17A and B

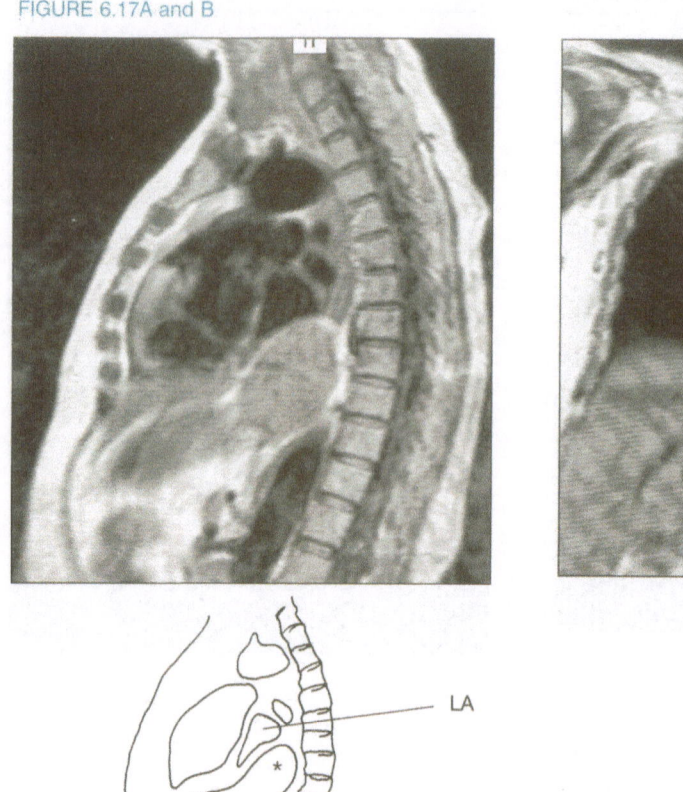

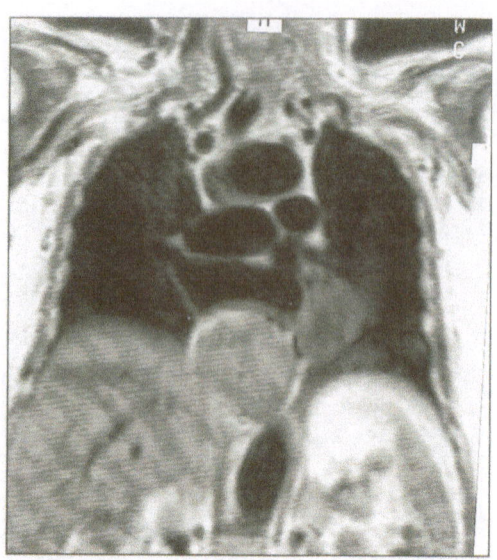

FIGURE 6.18

FIGURE 6.19

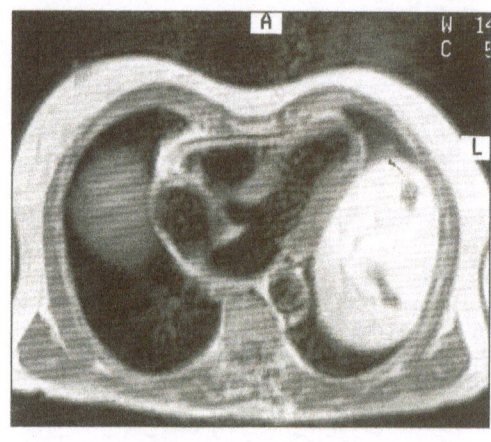

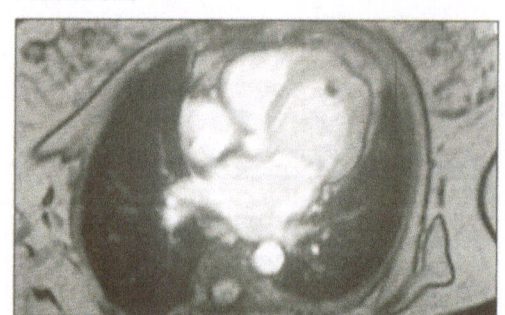

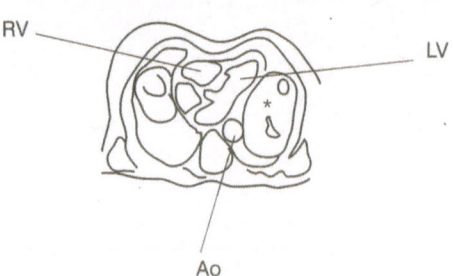

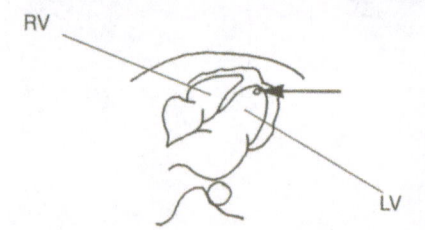

F. 6.17. Coronal (B) and sagittal (A) images which correspond to a hernia of the posterior segment of the right diaphragm that selectively compresses the left atrium and displaces the descending aorta (asterisk). Ao: aorta; LA: left atrium.

F. 6.18. T1 weighted spin echo axial image in which a deformation of the cardiac cavities due to the presence of two coexisting disorders is observed: pectus excavatum compressing anteriorly the right ventricle and an elevation of the left diaphragm (asterisk) compressing the left ventricle on its posterior aspect. Ao: aorta; LV: left ventricle; RV: right ventricle.

F. 6.19. Image from a gradient echo sequence corresponding to a patient with an old anteroseptal infarction and a mural thrombus (arrow) which stands out due to its low intensity signal. RV: right ventricle; LV: left ventricle.

8. Link KM, Lesko NM. MR evaluation of cardiac/juxtacardiac masses. Top Magn Reson Imaging 1995; 7: 232–45.

9. Hoffmann U, Globits S, Frank H. Cardiac and paracardiac masses. Current opinion on diagnostic evaluation by MRI. Eur Heart J 1998; 19: 553–63.

10. Mirowitz SA, Gutierrez FR. Fibromuscular elements of the right atrium: pseudomass at MR imaging. Radiology 1992; 182: 231–3.

11. Murphy MC, Sweeney MS, Putnam JB Jr, et al. Surgical treatment of cardiac tumors: a 25-year experience. Ann Thorac Surg 1990; 49: 612–8.

12. Lundt JT, Ehman RL, Julsrud PR, et al. Cardiac masses: assessment by MR imaging. Am J Roentgenol 1989; 152: 469–73.

13. Semelka RC, Shoenut JP, Wilson ME, Pellech AE, Patton JN. Cardiac masses: signal intensity features on spin-echo, gradient-echo, gadolinium-enhanced spin-echo, and turboFLASH images. J Magn Reson Imaging 1992; 2: 415–20.

14. Seelos KC, Funari M, Chang JM, Higgins ChB. Magnetic resonance imaging in acute and subacute mediastinal bleeding. Am Heart J 1992; 123: 1269–72.

15. Funari M, Fujita N, Peck WW, Higgins CB. Cardiac tumors: assessment with Gd-DTPA enhanced imaging. J Comput Assist Tomogr 1991; 15: 953–8.

16. Tazelaar HD, Locke TJ, McGregor CG. Pathology of surgically excised primary cardiac tumors. Mayo Clin Proc 1992; 67: 957–65.

17. Simon BC, Funck R, Drude L, Bohle RM, Reichart B, Maisch B. Malignant angiosarcoma of the right atrium in pregnancy. Diagnostic and therapeutic problems. Herz 1994; 19: 166–70.

18. Masauzi N, Ichikawa S, Nishimura F, et al. Primary angiosarcoma of the right atrium detected by magnetic resonance imaging. Intern Med 1992; 31: 1291–7.

19. Donatelli F, Pocar M, Moneta A, et al. Primary cardiac malignancy presenting as left atrial myxoma. Clinical and surgical considerations. Minerva Chir 1996 Jul–Aug;51(7–8): 585–8

20. White CS. MR evaluation of the pericardium and cardiac malignancies. Magn Reson Imaging Clin N Am 1996; 4: 237–51.

21. Hananouchi GI, Goff WB, 2d. Cardiac lipoma: six-year follow-up with MRI characteristics, and a review of the literature. Magn Reson Imaging 1990; 8(6): 825–8.

22. Hornero F, González I, Igual A et al. Hemangioma cardíaco primario. Presentación de un caso y revisión de la literatura. Rev Esp Cardiol 1993; 46: 509–11.

23. Burke AP, Rosado-de-Christenson M, Templeton PA, Virmani R. Cardiac fibroma: clinicopathologic correlates and surgical treatment. J Thorac Cardiovasc Surg 1994 Nov; 108(5): 862–70.

24. Tesoro-Tess JD, Biasi S, Balzarini L, et al. Heart involvement in lymphomas. The value of magnetic resonance imaging and two-dimensional echocardiography at disease presentation. Cancer 1993 Oct 15; 72(8): 2484–90

25. Gomes AS, Lois JF, Child JS. Cardiac tumors and thrombus: evaluation with MR imaging. Am J Radiol 1987; 149: 895.

26. Higgins CB, Caputo GR. Role of MR imaging in acquired and congenital cardiovascular disease. Am J Roentgenol 1993; 161: 13–22.

Diseases of the pericardium

7

G. PONS-LLADÓ

Introduction

The study of pericardial diseases is generally carried out satisfactorily by means of echocardiography. The detection of pericardial effusion was one of the first reported applications of the use of ultrasound[1]. Although the technique is totally accepted in clinical practice[2], its limitations in this field are recognized: there are limitations in the visualization of the anterior pericardium, in the estimation of the pericardial thickness and, in cases of pericardial effusion, problems arise when the process is localized or in the characterization of the nature of pericardial fluid.

Therefore, other imaging methods have been tested in the study of the pericardium. Computerized tomography has proven to be effective for obtaining useful images in pericardial effusion as well as in the detection of pericardial thickening or calcification[3]. The introduction of MRI has represented a significant advance due to its wide field of vision, its noninvasive nature and high resolution, with the possibility of characterizing fluid contents. The experience acquired with MRI has given the technique an outstanding role in the diagnosis of pericardial disorders, and at present it can be considered a resource of primary importance in this field.

7.1 The Normal Pericardium in Magnetic Resonance

In T1 spin echo sequences, the visceral and parietal components of the pericardium present as a regular curved line of low signal intensity due to the low hydrogen content of the fibrous tissue and to the small amount of fluid (15–50 ml) that is normally present between the layers of the pericardium. The visualization of this pericardial signal is in fact possible at sites where the presence of epicardial and paracardial adipose tissue, of high signal intensity, strongly contrasts with it and, thus, the pericardium is only clearly delineated at those levels in which some amount of neighboring fat is present, this occurring particularly in the anterior area, anterior to the right atrium and right ventricle (Figure 7.1). It is important to point out that the thickness of the pericardium determined in this way is normally 1–3 mm provided that the measurement is performed on diastolic images, since in systole the thickness may increase slightly[4]. It is also possible that apparently greater thickness due to tangential slicing may be seen in views at the level of the inferior aspect of the heart (see Figure 1.21)

7.2 Acute Pericarditis

Although the value of MR in the diagnosis of acute pericarditis has not been studied systematically, the technique is sensitive enough to detect percardiac thickening due to the inflammatory process[4,5]. In these cases, an increase in thickness of the pericardial space accompanied by an area of increased signal intensity due to inflammatory edema at this level is observed (Figure 7.2A) Although there is normally no clinical indication for routine MRI evaluation in simple acute pericarditis, the technique can be useful for follow-up studies in prolonged or recurrent cases (Figure 7.2B)

7.3 Pericardial Effusion

Although echocardiography is highly sensitive for the detection of pericardial effusion, the wide field of vision of MRI makes it superior in the visualization of localized processes, particularly in the posterior and apical regions, as well as for detecting the presence of associated pleural effusion[6].

In spin echo images, pericardial effusion presents as an increased pericardial space. This enlargement is not generally uniform, but it rather predominates in the posterior surface of the heart and in the lateral portions adjacent to the right atrium[5] (Figure 7.3)

The amount of the effusion determines the dimensions of the pericardial space in the MRI views. It is accepted that a space larger than 5 mm between the anterior right ventricle and the parietal pericardium just beneath the anterior chest wall is indicative of a moderate degree of effusion[5]. Nevertheless, experimental studies have shown[7] that although the technique detects the presence of an infusion of pericardiac fluid of 5 ml, there is a considerable overlap of the dimensions of the effusion when the quantity of injected fluids oscillates between 40 and 120 ml, volumes which, in practical terms, would represent degrees of moderate and important effusion, respectively.

The ability of MR to characterize fluid contents is useful for estimating the type of pericardiac effusion: signal intensity will be low for serofibrinous types[5] (Figure 7.3) intermediate for the exudates[6] (Figure 7.4) and high for the hemopericardium[8] (Figure 7.5), although it has been demonstrated experimentally[7] that signals of similar intensity can occur in the last two cases. This extreme sensitivity of MRI means that areas of different signal intensity are observed in the interior of the effusion. In serous effusions, regions with a slight increase in intensity are frequently observed, which indicates the presence of a high level of proteins and cellular elements that, due to the effect of gravity, produce sediment in the lower portions of the effusion, which suggests an inflammatory nature[4,6] (Figure 7.3).

The presence of an apparent increase in the anterior pericardiac space, without being accompanied by a posterior effusion, is frequently a cause of a false-positive diagnosis of pericardial effusion in echocardiographic studies. In these cases, MRI generally reveals the presence of a prominent adipose pad[9], which permits the diagnosis of pericardial effusion to be excluded (Figure 7.6)

7.4 Constrictive Pericarditis

The recognized difficulties involved in the clinical distinction between constrictive pericarditis and restrictive cardiomyopathy justify the use of a technique that permits a reliable differential diagnosis between the two entities.

In spin echo images, pericardial constriction is characterized by an increase in the width of the low intensity signal of the

FIGURE 7.1

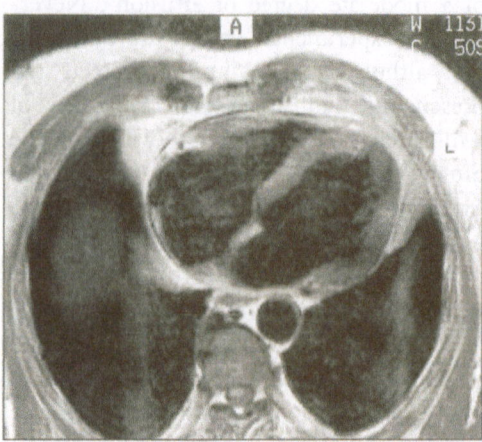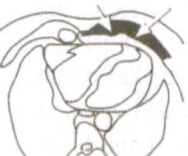

FIGURE 7.2 A and B

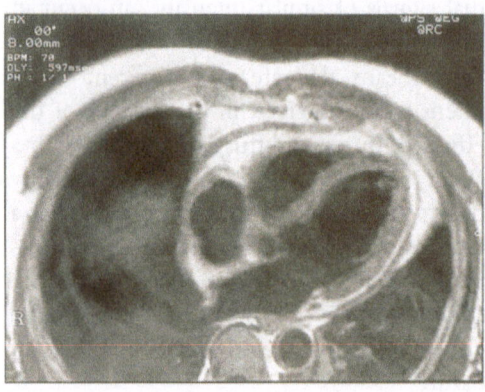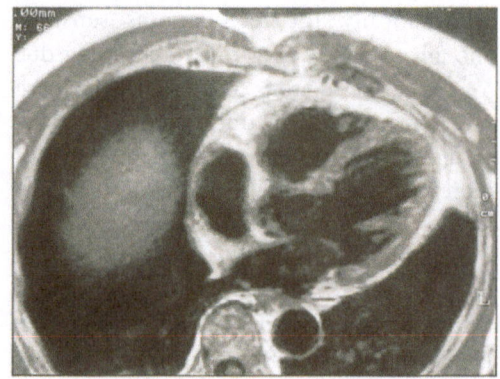

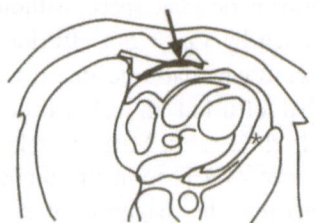

F. 7.1.　Axial plane showing the linear signal of low intensity corresponding to the normal pericardium (arrows). In this case a considerable extension of the pericardium is observed due to the presence of abundant epicardial and paracardial fat, their high signal intensity facilitating the contrast with the pericardium.

F. 7.2.　(A) Axial plane in a patient with recurrent acute pericarditis obtained during an episode of relapse: a diffuse pericardial thickening is observed (arrow), as well as an increase in signal intensity in the posterior parietal pericardium (asterisk); (B) Plane at the same level obtained 6 months later after remission of symptoms: the pericardium presents a practically normal MRI appearance.

F. 7.3.　Axial plane in a case of pericardial effusion (arrows). Note the area of slightly higher signal intensity in the posterior pericardial cavity, which indicates an effusion content rich in protein and cellular elements.

F. 7.4.　Axial plane showing pericardial effusion (arrow) with a signal of intermediate intensity corresponding to a chronic pericarditis of tuberculous origin. Bilateral pleural effusion is also present.

F. 7.5.　Axial plane that depicts the presence of pericardial effusion localized on the posterior surface (arrow) in a patient who had undergone coronary bypass surgery. The high signal intensity of the effusion suggests a hematic content.

F. 7.6.　Sagittal plane that depicts a signal of the normal pericardium (arrow), although with a marked epicardial adipose pad (asterisk). Its high signal intensity contrasts with the low signal of the pericardium as well as with the intermediate one of the myocardium of the right ventricle.

FIGURE 7.3

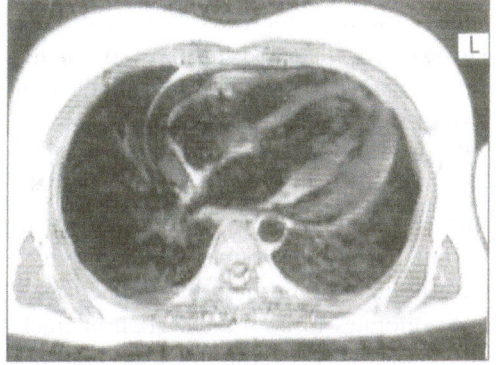

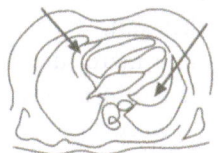

FIGURE 7.5

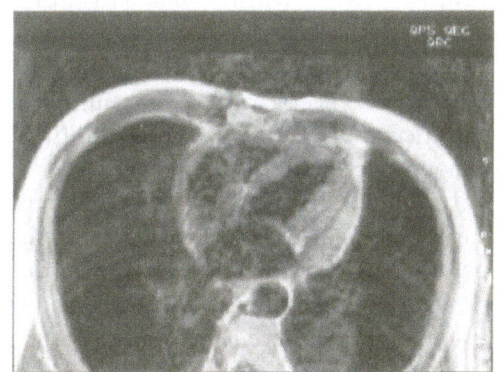

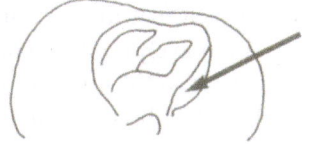

FIGURE 7.4

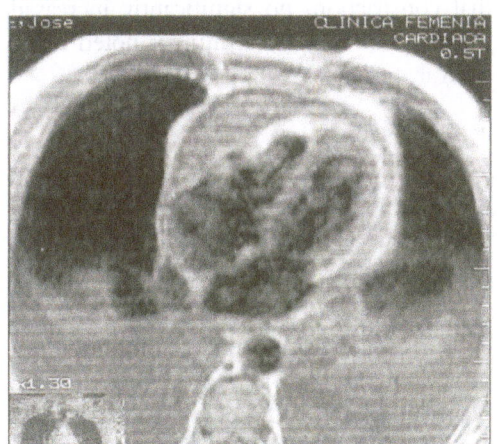

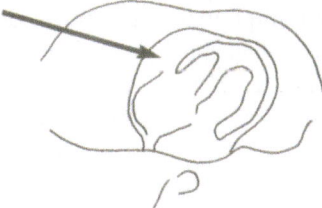

FIGURE 7.6

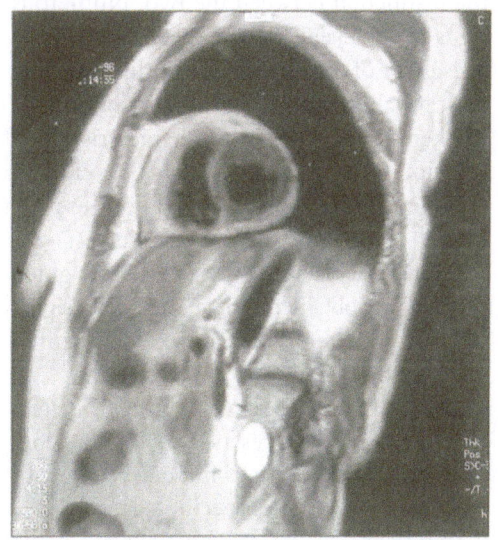

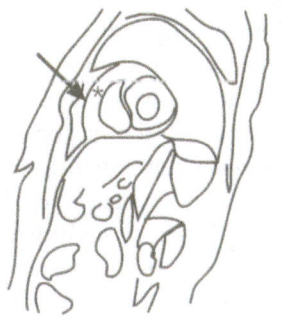

pericardium due its thickened fibrous component (Figure 7.7). When an additional inflammatory component exists, an epicardial zone with increased signal intensity also appears[8] (Figure 7.8). Pericardiac thickening in constrictive pericarditis is typically diffuse, although not uniform[10,11]. Frequently, it is only observed in determined regions, particularly in the anterior aspect since, in the posterior segments, the absence of epicardial fat frequently prevents an adequate delimitation of the thickened pericardium.

The value of pericardial thickness that is considered indicative of abnormal thickening is 4 mm, provided that the measurement is not taken in excessively basal (diaphragmatic) slices of the heart and that images in systole are avoided, as has been stated above. By using this criteria, sensitivity values of 88% and specificity of 100% for the diagnosis of constriction have been reported[11].

The fact that pericardial thickening and the presence of effusion both present a low signal intensity in the spin-echo technique compels the distinction between the two. Numerous signs of thickening have been noted: the presence of an irregular outline in the pericardial image; a signal distribution of thickening that is not characteristic of effusion, as has been noted previously, including the lack of occupation of the pericardial recesses in the great vessels[5] (Figure 7.9); and the fact that when T2 weighted images are obtained, the pericardiac signal intensity does not increase, as opposed to what is observed in the case of effusion[11].

One aspect that deserves comment is that, as is known, the presence of calcification, pericardial in this case, is not detectable with MRI, as an area of nonspecific signal absence is observed (Figure 7.10), which may on the other hand contribute to the above-mentioned irregularity of the outlines of the thickened pericardium. Owing to this, a sign that has been traditionally considered to be one of the most specific of constriction is lost, one to which conventional radiological techniques are very sensitive. From a practical point of view, nevertheless, this limitation must be considered to be relative, since it has been noted that the presence of calcification of the pericardium is now less prevalent than before in patients with clinical symptoms of pericardial constriction[12].

Other signs that can be observed in an MRI study in constrictive pericarditis are the tubular morphology of the ventricular chambers, a flattened form of the interventricular wall and dilatation of the right atrium and the inferior vena cava (Figure 7.11). All these contribute to the hemodynamic alteration caused by constriction, and all are indirect signs that can be modified by eventual medical treatment and, therefore, have limited diagnostic value[11]. The crucial fact continues to be the detection of thickening of the pericardium, a finding that permits restrictive cardiomyopathy to be effectively ruled out. Nevertheless, and importantly, the mere detection of an increased pericardial thickness does not equal constriction[10,11], since it can be seen in situations such as those following cardiac surgery[13] or in the evolutive course of a simple pericarditis without clinical manifestations of congestion (Figure 7.2). On the other hand, it has been reported that in between 10%[11] and 20%[5] of cases of pericardial constriction, no significantly increased thickness of the pericardium is noted using MRI (Figure 7.12).

7.5 Congenital Pericardial Diseases

An infrequent abnormality, although an important one due to the differential diagnostic problems it originates, is the *congenital absence of the pericardium*. It is frequently partial and affects the left portion, the patients being generally asymptomatic. It is usually detected in the form of an apparent cardiomegaly in a chest x-ray, and even though there are specific signs in the outline of the cardiac silhouette that cause suspicion, confirmation of the diagnosis is always recommended, for which MR is useful[14]. Although the simple lack of signal corresponding to the pericardium in MR images is not of value, since, as has been noted, it is frequently not visualized in all its extension, there are demonstrative signs of its congenital absence. They consist of the displacement of the cardiac cavities, which are otherwise normal with respect to their dimensions while the

FIGURE 7.7

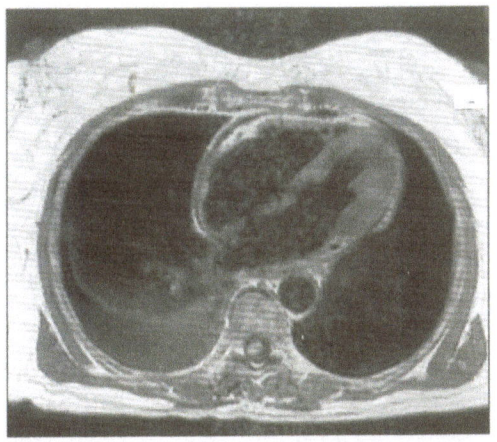

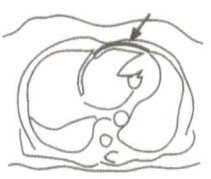

FIGURE 7.8

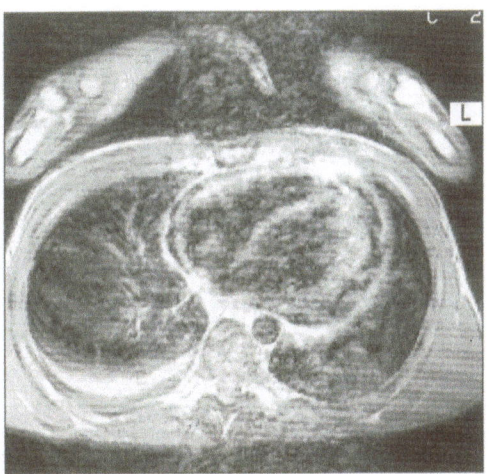

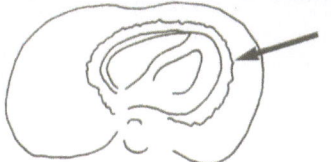

FIGURE 7.9 A and B

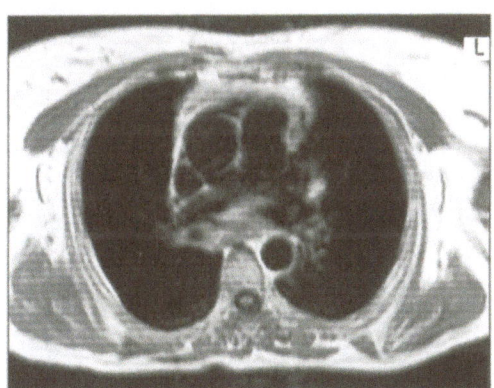

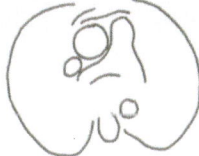

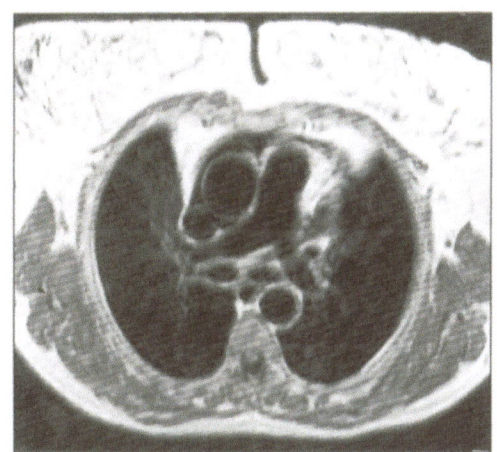

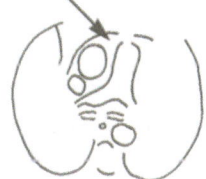

F. 7.7.   Pericardial thickening (arrows) in a case of constrictive pericarditis.

F. 7.8.   Pericardial effusion and thickening of the membrane with an increase in signal intensity (arrow) in a case of
tuberculous pericarditis (compare with Figure 7.3).

F. 7.9.   Axial planes at the level of the great vessels in the same patient obtained in supine (A) and prone (B) positions: an
enlargement of the pre-aortic pericardial sinus is observed in B (arrow) due to the displacement of the pericardial
content in the prone position, this proving the presence of pericardial effusion.

FIGURE 7.10

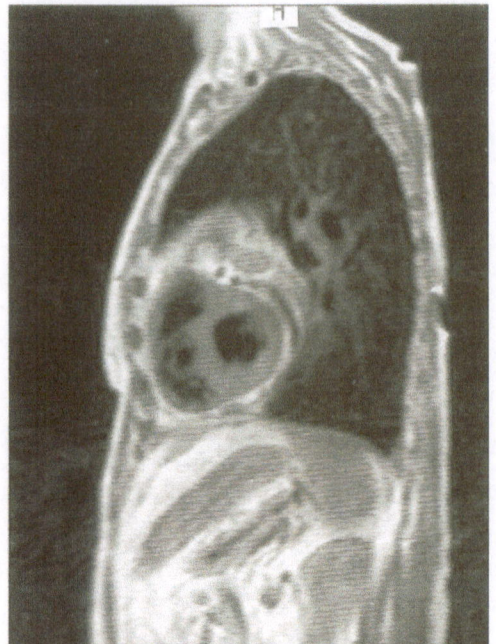

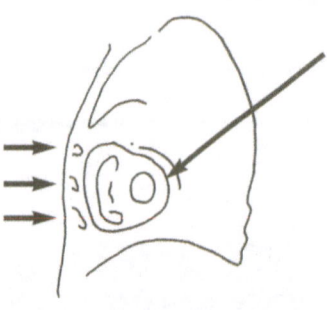

FIGURE 7.11

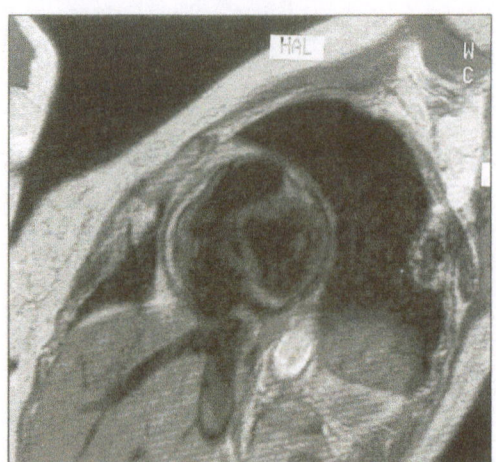

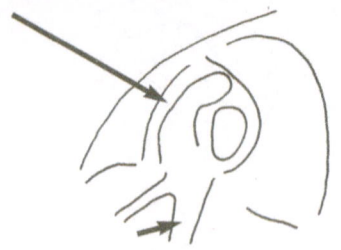

FIGURE 7.12

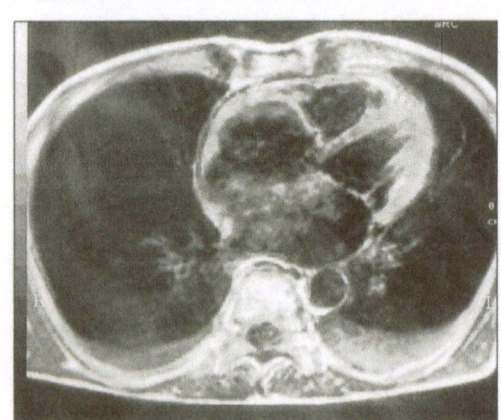

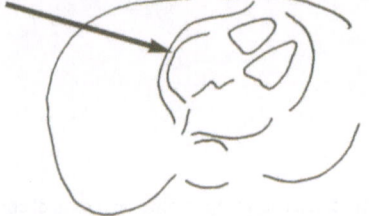

F. 7.10. Sagittal plane in a case of calcified constrictive pericarditis where, in addition to a thickened pericardium at the posterior aspect of the heart (large arrow), areas of absent signal in the anterior aspect (short arrows) are also seen probably due to calcinous foci.

F. 7.11. Oblique sagittal plane in a case of constrictive pericarditis showing a thickened pericardium (large arrows) and a dilatation of the inferior vena cava and hepatic vein (short arrow)

F. 7.12. Axial plane showing only mild thickening of the pericardium (arrow) in a patient with overt clinical signs of constriction which was later proven at surgery.

extrapericardial structures, such as the great vessels, maintain their normal position (Figure 7.13). On one hand, correct identification of this alteration is important in order to rule out other causes of radiological cardiomegaly, and, on the other hand, in order to identify those forms of congenital absence of the pericardium with possible risk of strangulation of the cardiac structures[15], which require surgical treatment. It must likewise be kept in mind that up to 30% of the cases involving absence of the pericardium are associated with other intracardiac congenital malformations[16].

The *pericardial cyst* is a benign lesion that originates during embryonic development of the pericardium and which is frequently asymptomatic. It is normally detected due to a deformed cardiac silhouette in a chest x-ray, and is often located in the right anterior cardiophrenic region. Its clear fluid content and sharp definition of its edges cause the images to be always demonstrative. Adjacent to the heart, a mass with typical cystic characteristics is observed, which has a round or ovoid form and a low or intermediate signal intensity in its interior in T1 spin echo sequences (Figure 7.14), which increases homogeneously in T2 images[16]. The study of the signal intensity of the interior of the mass can help to distinguish the pericardial cyst from other mediastinal lesions, such as thymic or bronchogenic cysts, where it is more frequent to find a high signal intensity due to the presence of hemorrhage[17].

References

1. Feigenbaum H, Waldhausen JA, Hyde LP. Ultrasound diagnosis of pericardial effusion. J Am Med Assoc (JAMA) 1965; 191: 107–10.

2. Chandraratna PAN. Echocardiography and Doppler ultrasound in the evaluation of pericardial disease. Circulation 1991; 84 (Suppl. I): I-303–I-310.

3. Silverman PM, Harell GS. Computed tomography of the normal pericardium. Invest Radiol 1983; 18: 141–4.

4. Stark DD, Higgins CB, Lanzer P, et al. Magnetic resonance imaging of the pericardium : normal and pathologic findings. Radiology 1984; 150: 469–74.

5. Sechtem U, Tscholakoff D, Higgins CB. MRI of the abnormal pericardium. Am J Roentgenol 1986; 147: 245–52.

6. Mulvagh SL, Rokey R, Vick III GW, Johnston DL. Usefulness of nuclear magnetic resonance imaging for the evaluation of pericardial effusions, and comparison with two-dimensional echocardiography. Am J Cardiol 1989; 64: 1002–9.

7. Rokey R, Vick III GW, Bolli R, Lewandowski ED. Assessment of experimental pericardial effusion using nuclear magnetic resonance imaging techniques. Am Heart J 1991; 121: 1161–9.

8. Germain Ph, Kastler B, Baruthio J, et al. Magnetic resonance imaging in pericardial pathology. Echocardiography 1989; 6: 203–11.

9. Duvernoy O, Larsson SG, Thuren J, Rauschning W. Epicardial fat causing pitfalls in CT and MR imaging of the pericardium. Acta Radiol 1992; 33: 1–5.

10. Soulen RL, Stark DD, Higgins CB. Magnetic resonance imaging of constrictive pericardial disease. Am J Cardiol 1985; 55: 480–4.

11. Masui T, Finck S, Higgins CB. Constrictive pericarditis and restrictive cardiomyopathy: evaluation with MR imaging. Radiology 1992; 182: 369–73.

12. Vaitkus PT, Kussmaul WG. Constrictive pericarditis versus restrictive cardiomyopathy: a reappraisal and update of diagnostic criteria. Am Heart J 1991; 122: 1431–41.

13. Duvernoy O, Malm T, Thuomas KA, Larsson SG, Hansson HE. CT and MR evaluation of pericardial and retrosternal adhesions after cardiac surgery. J Comput Assist Tomogr 1991; 15: 555–60.

14. Altman CA, Ettedgui JA, Wozney P, Beerman LB. Noninvasive diagnostic features of partial absence of the pericardium. Am J Cardiol 1989; 63: 1536–7.

15. Gassner I, Judmaier W, Fink C, et al. Diagnosis of congenital pericardial defects, including a pathognomic sign for dangerous apical ventricular herniation, on magnetic resonance imaging. Br Heart J 1995; 74: 60–6.

16. White CS. MR evaluation of the pericardium and cardiac malignancies. Magn Reson Imaging Clin N Am 1996; 4: 237–52.

17. Murayama S, Murakami J, Watanabe H, et al. Signal intensity characteristics of mediastinal cystic masses on T1 weighted MRI. J Comput Assist Tomogr 1995; 19: 188–91.

FIGURE 7.13 A and B

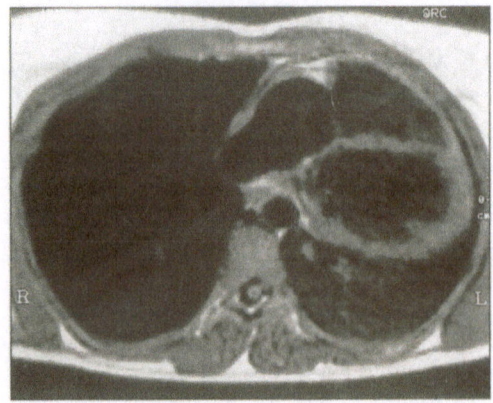 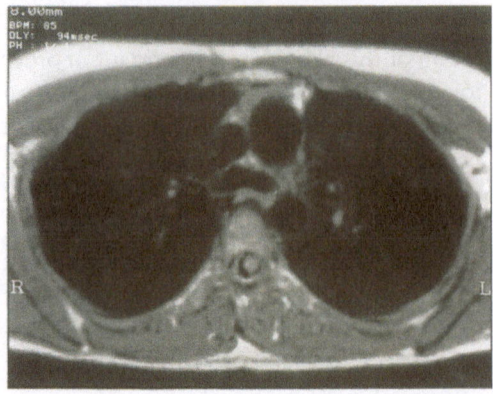

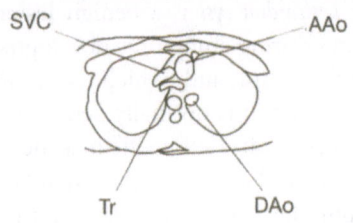

FIGURE 7.14

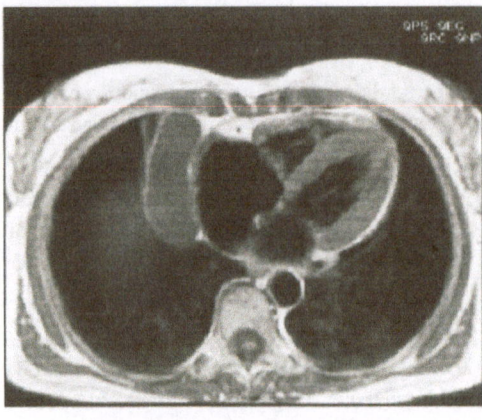

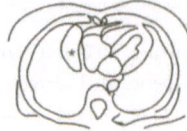

F. 7.13. (A) Axial plane at the ventricular level in a case of partial agenesis of the left pericardium. Note the displacement of the heart toward the left hemithorax in the absence of a thoracic cause, the cardiac chambers being otherwise normal in size. (B) High thoracic plane in the same case that displays a normal position in the mediastinum of the extrapericardial structures. AAo: ascending aorta; DAo: descending aorta; SVC: superior vena cava; Tr: trachea.

F. 7.14. Axial plane that depicts a pericardial cyst (asterisk) adjacent to the right atrium, a characteristic position of this type of lesion, with a low or intermediate signal intensity in its interior suggesting a serous fluid content.

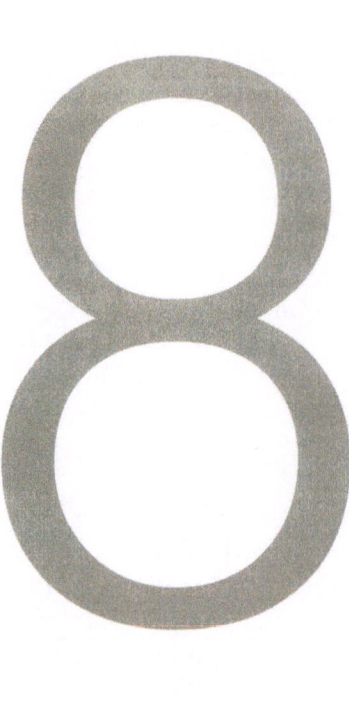

Congenital heart disease 8

M. SUBIRANA-DOMÉNECH
X. BORRÁS-PÉREZ

Introduction

Magnetic resonance imaging (MRI) is an extremely useful tool to study congenital heart disease as it has the main advantages of both echocardiography and conventional angiography[1,2,3]. Like echocardiography, MRI is a noninvasive technique providing accurate morphological information on the heart and, as angiography, it allows the study of extracardiac vascular structures. This latter characteristic is very important, because it permits evaluation of the ventriculo-arterial connections, the position and relationship between the great arteries and the drainage of the systemic and pulmonary veins[4]. An additional advantage of MRI that should be noted is its excellent image quality in the majority of patients, including adults[5] and those who have been submitted to surgical cardiac correction, as it does not require a particular window to obtain images[6], neither has it limitations in the orientation of views, and it can produce images in any desired plane of the heart[7].

8.1 Segmental Study of Congenital Heart Disease

In the study of congenital anomalies of the heart and the great vessels the description of the localization and morphology of the different cardiovascular structures as well as the existing connections between them is very important. This is known as segmental analysis of the heart. The diagnosis of cardiac malpositions and of the *situs* can be approached using radiology, electrocardiography or echocardiography, but the study of venous drainage, atrioventricular and ventriculoarterial connections as well as the relative position of the different cardiac segments, especially in the case of complex cardiac anomalies, is more easily carried out by MRI.

8.2 Study of Atria and Venous Connections

The first step consists of the assessment of the position and orientation of the heart within the thoracic cavity (levocardia, dextrocardia or mesocardia) (Figure 8.1). The following step is the determination of the atrial *situs*. The morphologically right atrium is normally located anteriorly and to the right. It is characterized by a triangular-shaped atrial appendage with a wide connection to the rest of the atrium. The morphologically left atrium has smoother walls and an appendage that is narrower and finger-like shaped. The situation where a morphologically right atrium is situated to the right of a morphologically left atrium (normal position) is known as atrial *situs solitus* (Figure 8.2). When the morphologically left atrium is placed anterior and to the right of a morphologically right atrium, it is known as atrial *situs inversus*. When both atria have similar morphology (both right or both left), it is known as atrial *isomerism* (right or left respectively) and the *situs* is called *situs ambiguus*. MRI has shown a high capacity to determine the atrial and thoracic *situs*, since segmental anatomy is optimally displayed in transverse and coronal planes. By MRI spin echo it is possible to identify the morphologically left and right atrium as well as the left and the right main bronchi. It is of great help, because usually there is a spatial concordance between those structures, atrium and bronchi. Likewise, as a consequence of its wide field of view, MRI also allows the analysis of the abdominal *situs*,[8] which is generally concordant with the atrial and thoracic *situs*. In case of discordance between the atrial and the visceral *situs*, the diagnosis of *situs ambiguus* should be suspected; it is almost always associated with the asplenia (right atrial isomerism) or polysplenia (left atrial isomerism) syndromes.

Systemic venous blood return can help in assessing the atrial *situs*. In *situs solitus*, the inferior vena cava is located to the right of the vertebral column and drains into a morphologically right atrium, placed on the right. In *situs inversus*, the inferior vena cava is located to the left of the vertebral column and drains into a morphologically right atrium, placed on the left. In cases of *situs ambiguus*, associated with a syndrome of polysplenia, the suprahepatic veins usually drain directly into the atrium. The syndrome is characterized by two morphologically left atria, two long main bronchi (morphologically left), a central liver, multiple spleens and interruption of the inferior vena cava with continuation of the abdominal venous blood return through the system of the azygos or hemiazygos veins. In *situs ambiguus* associated with a syndrome of asplenia, the two atrial cavities are morphologically right, the two main bronchi are short (morphologically right), the liver is placed in the middle of the abdominal cavity, there is no spleen and the inferior vena cava and the abdominal aorta are usually situated on the same side of the vertebral column with the vein in an antero-lateral position. By using axial, coronal and sagittal slices, the location, course and flow of the inferior vena cava can be observed by MRI. It is a very useful technique not only for identifying situs but also for the study of the anomalies of systemic venous return. In case of interruption of the inferior vena cava, the level of interruption and the venous abdominal return through the azygos and hemiazygos veins can be detected, especially using coronal planes. Likewise, a direct drainage of suprahepatic veins into the atrium can be easily displayed (Figure 8.3).

The superior vena cava usually drains into a morphologically right atrium. A dilated superior vena cava suggests either an anomaly causing systemic venous hypertension, or an obstruction of the drainage of this vein (Figure 8.4).

A frequent anomaly of the systemic venous return is a persistent left superior vena cava, that generally drains into a dilated coronary sinus. It may be easily diagnosed by MRI (Figure 8.5).

The coronary sinus is seen in axial planes behind the morphologically left atrium. As has been noted previously, a dilatated coronary sinus suggests as a first diagnostic option a persistent left superior vena cava; however, it may be seen in cases of anomalous drainage of the pulmonary veins or arteriovenous fistula draining into it.

The four pulmonary veins drain into the left atrium through its posterior wall and can be easily visualized by using both the

FIGURE 8.1

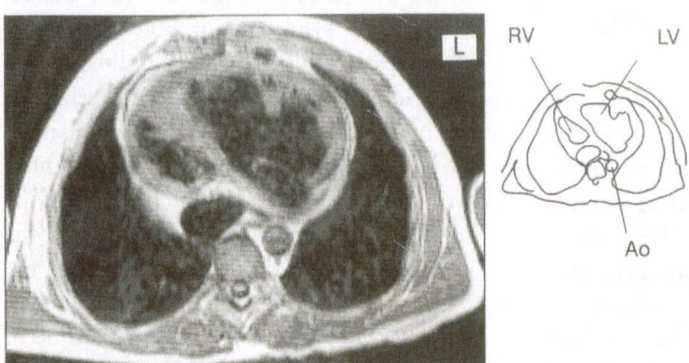

FIGURE 8.2A and B

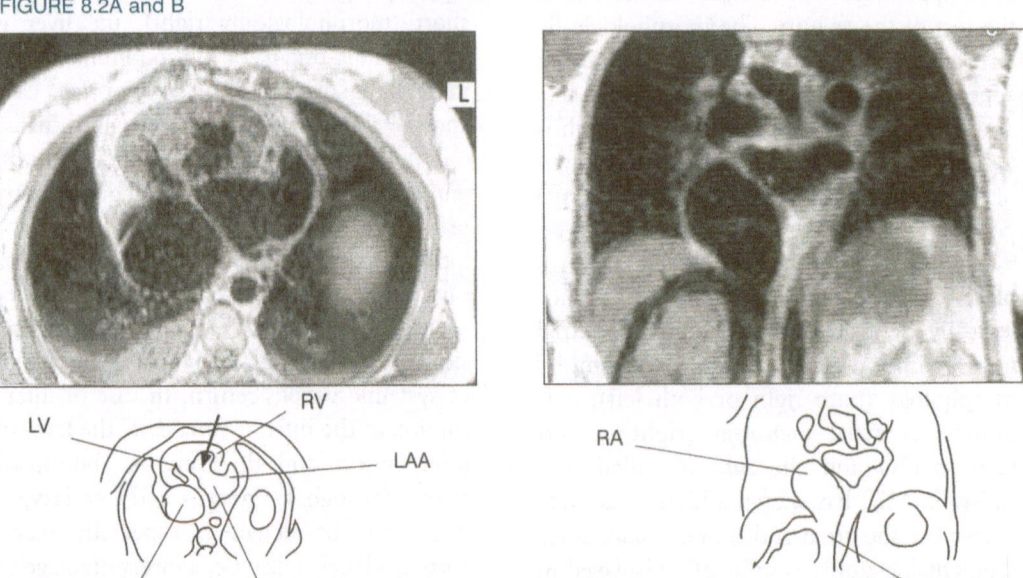

FIGURE 8.3A and B

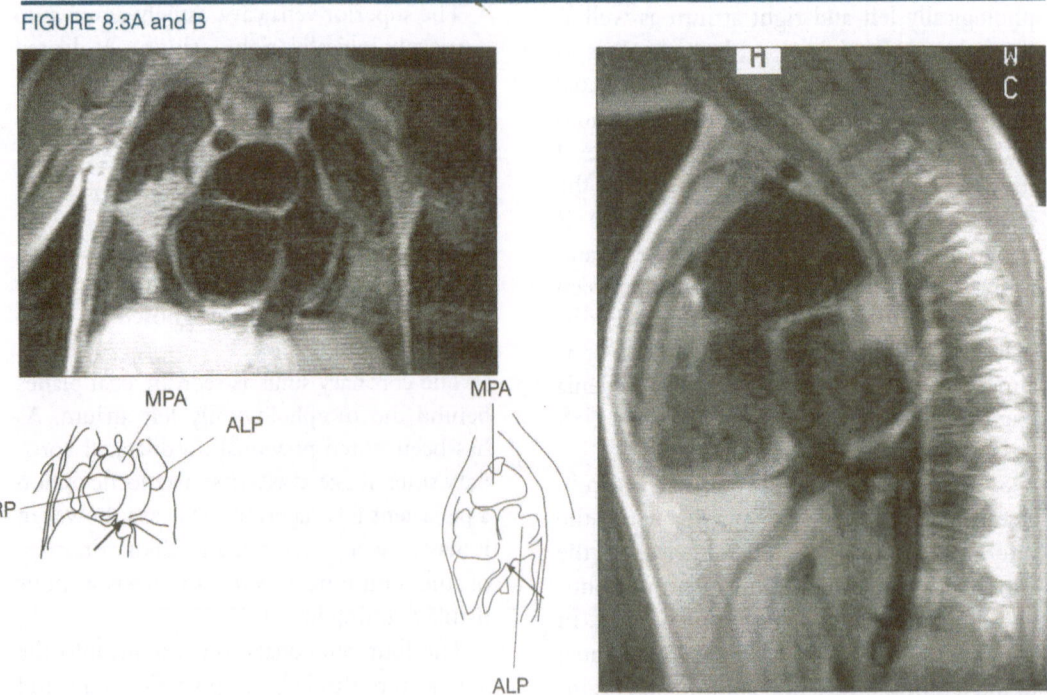

FIGURE 8.4A and B

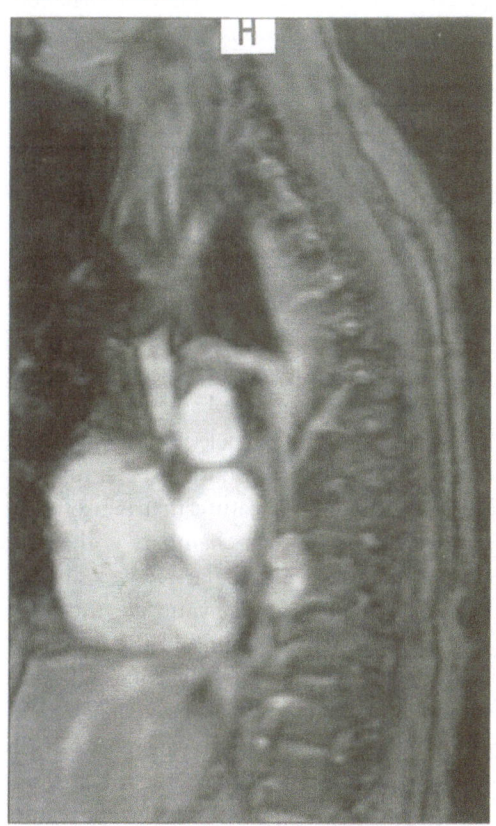

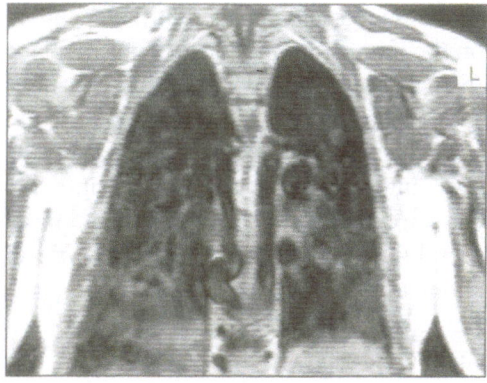

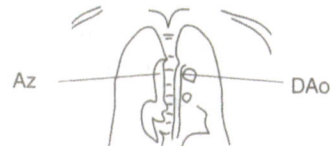

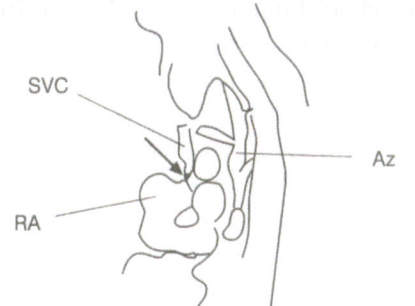

F. 8.1.   Axial slice showing a heart in mesocardia with the apex directed toward the right side of the thorax (dextroversion) in a patient diagnosed with double outlet left ventricle. Ao: aorta; LV: left ventricle; RV: right ventricle.

F. 8.2.   (A) Axial plane showing: a) the heart placed on the right side within the chest (dextrocardia) with the apex directed toward the right (dextroversion), b) the morphologically left atrial appendage (digitiform) situated on the left, and c) the septal insertion of the atrioventricular valve placed on the left, closer to the the apex (arrow) than the other one placed on the right; then, it is morphologically right, and consequently the ventricle may be identified as morphologically right, by the rule that the atrio-ventricular valve always belongs to the appropiate ventricle. (B) Coronal plane that shows an inferior vena cava, situated on the right, draining into an atrium placed on the right, suggesting the diagnosis of situs solitus. The study shows a patient affected by a complex congenital heart disease with dextrocardia, dextroversion, situs solitus and atrioventricular discordance. IVC: inferior vena cava; LA: left atrium; LAA: left atrial appendage; LV: left ventricle; RA: right atrium; RV: right ventricle.

F. 8.3.   (A) Coronal and (B) sagittal planes showing the direct drainage of the suprahepatic veins (arrow) into an atrial cavity, which, as is shown in the coronal slice, is situated on the left. Note the dilated pulmonary arterial trunk, practically aneurysmatic. This is a child with left atrial isomerism and the heart placed in the middle of the chest (mesocardia). ALP: atrium in left position; ARP: atrium in right position; MPA: main pulmonary artery.

F. 8.4.   Obstruction of the superior vena cava after surgical closure with a patch of a sinus venosus atrial septal defect situated near the entry of this vessel. (A) Sagittal plane in gradient echo technique showing the severe stenosis (arrow) at level of the drainage of the vena cava into the atrium. The alternative venous drainage toward the azygos vein is also shown. (B) Coronal plane in spin echo showing collateral circulation through the azygos vein system. AV: azygos vein; DAo: descending aorta; RA: right atrium; SVC: superior vena cava.

spin echo and the gradient echo MRI techniques. There are different types of anomalies of the pulmonary venous return, depending on the number of pulmonary veins involved (partial or total anomalous pulmonary venous connection) and on the draining structure (into the right atrium, into the superior vena cava, into the inferior vena cava, into the coronary sinus, etc.). MRI is much more useful than echocardiography to diagnose an anomalous pulmonary venous drainage (sensitivity: 95% versus 38%), being even superior to angiography (sensitivity: 69%)[9]. Axial planes are usually enough to diagnose the anomaly, but in some cases the use of additional sagittal or coronal planes may be necessary (Figure 8.6). The identification of any one of the four pulmonary veins draining into the left atrium excludes the diagnosis of a total anomalous pulmonary connection.

The *sinus venosus* type of atrial septal defect is frequently associated with a partial anomalous pulmonary venous drainage. The right superior pulmonary vein drains into the right atrium or the superior vena cava. In the latter case, using axial planes a defect is observed in the lateral wall of the superior vena cava, a typical image that has been described as the sign of the "broken ring."[10]

In total anomalous pulmonary venous drainage (TAPVD), the pulmonary veins usually converge in a common collector. It may drain at supradiaphragmatic level, either into intracardiac structures (coronary sinus, right atrium) or into extracardiac ones (right superior vena cava, azygos vein, innominate vein, left superior vena cava), or at infradiaphragmatic level (inferior vena cava or portal system). This last situation is usually associated with an obstruction of the pulmonary venous return and as a consequence, with pulmonary venous hypertension. The wide field of view of MRI allows visualization of the complete courses of TPAVD, including pulmonary veins, pulmonary venous confluences, vertical veins, and entrance of the vertical veins, usually providing all that is needed for the diagnosis. However, as this abnormality presents with early clinical symptoms, the diagnosis is usually achieved by echocardiography, MRI being more useful in the postoperative control of these patients. It may help to detect some residual lesions or sequelae

requiring a further surgical intervention (5–20 % of the cases)[11], such as obstruction of the pulmonary venous return.[12]

8.3   Atrioventricular Connections

The ventricles may be identified on the basis of their morphology and on the anatomical characteristics of the atrioventricular valves. The right ventricle usually displays a triangular form, with a coarse trabecular pattern and with the moderator band situated near the apex. The left ventricle presents with an elliptical form with a smoother septal surface. Another anatomical feature that is useful in identifying the cardiac chambers is the fact that the atrio-ventricular valve always belongs to the appropriate ventricle; thus, the mitral valve is always found in the morphologically left ventricle, and the tricuspid valve in the morphologically right ventricle. We can identify the tricuspid valve because it inserts in the interventricular septum closer to the apex than the mitral valve, and because it has chordal insertions into the ventricular septum. The mitral valve has chordal insertions into two papillary muscles and is a bicuspid valve, fish-mouth shaped.

Atrioventricular concordance describes the situation where of the morphologically right atrium is connected to the morphologically right ventricle and the morpholgically left atrium to the morphologically left ventricle. The connection is called discordant when the morphologically right atrium connects to the morphologically left ventricle and the morphologically left atrium connects to the morphologically right ventricle, independently of the spatial position of the chambers (Figure 8.2A). In cases of atrial isomerism the atrioventricular connection is known as ambiguous. There are other types of atrioventricular connections, as when the two atria connect directly to a single ventricle (double inlet atrio-ventricular connection) and when only one atrium is connected to a ventricular inlet portion. In the latter arrangement, the other atrioventricular connection is absent (tricuspid or mitral atresia). Because of this, a rudimentary ventricular chamber may be present, which does not receive an inlet portion. Some authors group hearts with double inlet or with absence on one atrioventricular connection together as univentricular hearts.

The type of atrioventricular connection (concordant, discordant, ambiguous, double inlet and absent right or left) should be differentiated from the mode of atrioventricular connection. The mode describes the specific morphology of the valve apparatus and may occur with any type of connection. When there are two atrioventricular connection, these may be through two patent atrioventricular valves, through a common atrioventricular valve, or through the the combination of a permeable valve and an imperforate valve. At the same time an incorrect alignment of the connection may exist (valve in overriding or straddling position).

MRI is an useful technique to study the atrioventricular connections, especially by using the axial planes in the spin echo sequences. In some cases of complex anomalies it may be necessary to use projections with a different obliquity instead of the standard tomographic planes. One of the limitations of the technique is its suboptimal resolution in the visualization of valves as they are thin and move rapidly, not being easily visible by MRI. Then, some valvular abnormalities such as mitral or tricuspid valve prolapse, myxoid degeneration, clefts, imperforation, etc., are better studied by echocardiography.

8.4 Ventriculoarterial Connections

When the pulmonary artery originates from a morphologically right ventricle and the aorta arises from a morphologically left ventricle (more than 50% of the sigmoid annulus arising from the ventricular chamber), the ventriculoarterial connection is called concordant. When the morphologically left ventricle connects to the pulmonary artery and the morphologically right ventricle to the aorta, a ventriculoarterial discordance occurs, independently from the spatial position of the different chambers and/or vessels. The

term "transposition" should be reserved for defining a type of relationship of the great vessels and it is important to remember that any relationship may occur with any arterial connection. In a normal anatomical pattern, the aorta is placed posterior and to the left of the pulmonary artery, and the outflow tract of the right ventricle is wrapped anteriorly around the left ventricular outflow tract and aortic root. When the aorta is situated in a position anterior to the pulmonary artery then the great vessels are in transposition, L-transposition occurring when the aorta is anterior and to the left of the pulmonary artery, and D-transposition when it is placed anterior and to the right of the pulmonary artery. These arteries are identified according to the presence or absence of bifurcation: the pulmonary arterial trunk rapidly bifurcates into two pulmonary branches, while the aorta does not.

In contrast to echocardiography, MRI has no restrictions in the acquisition of views of the great vessels. This usually allows their easy identification, study of their relationship and description of the type of ventriculoarterial connection. Likewise, it permits the evaluation of the size of the aorta and the pulmonary arteries[13], including the main and the distal pulmonary arteries, and may be especially useful in diagnosing branch pulmonary artery discontinuity and stenosis, which is very important in the evaluation of surgical possibilities.

To visualize the pulmonary artery bifurcation (the clue for its identification), MRI axial planes of the thorax are usually the most useful (Figure 8.7). They also provide information about the position of the ascending aorta, normally placed posterior and to the right of the pulmonary artery, and of the descending aorta, which under normal conditions runs along the left side of the vertebral column. Coronal planes are generally useful for the study of the ascending aorta and the aortic arch branches. Mild angulations of these planes may improve the visualization of these structures. Cine-MRI technique permits the study of blood flow conditions and detection of possible anomalies in it. Additionally, the velocity mapping technique can be used to measure the flow into different vascular structures.

FIGURE 8.5A and B

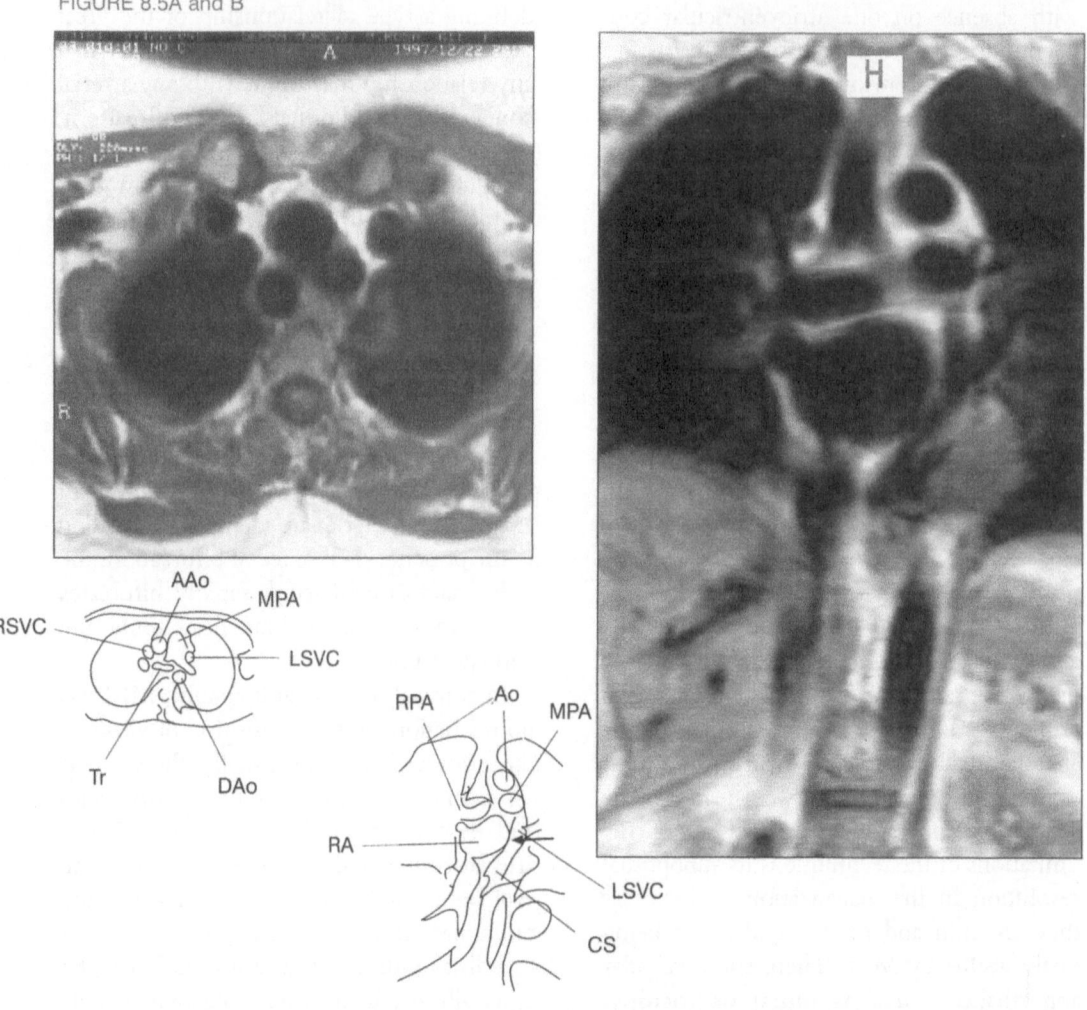

FIGURE 8.6

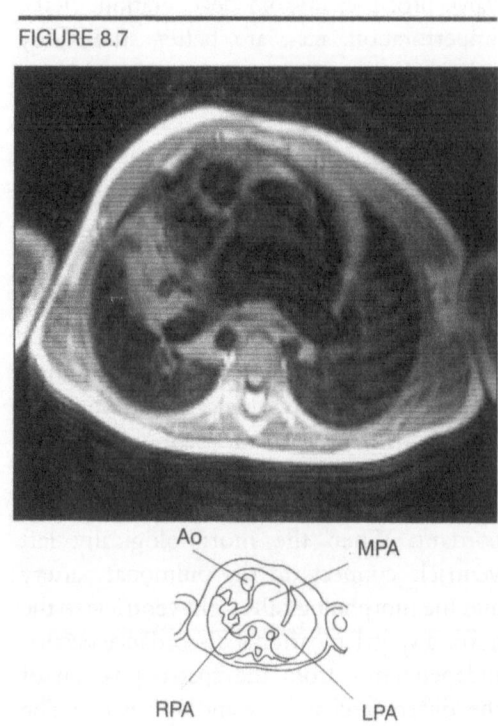

FIGURE 8.7

8.5 Study of Shunts

A frequent abnormality in congenital heart disease is the presence of a communication between the systemic and the pulmonary circulation, producing a shunt. Usually, the shunt is left-to-right causing an increase in pulmonary flow. The shunt can be isolated or associated with other congenital anomalies, in which case the shunting of blood can be essential for the survival of the patient, as occurs in cases of congenital dependent ductus arteriosus.

The study of shunts requires an appropriate assessment of: 1) the morphology, size and position (atrial, ventricular, great vessels, etc.) of the defect, 2) the direction and volume of the shunt, and 3) its hemodynamic overload on the heart. The most frequent shunts can be found in the following malformations: atrial septal defect, ventricular septal defect and patent ductus arteriosus. Other shunts may be the result of an anomalous pulmonary venous drainage, an aortopulmonary window or an arteriovenous fistula. The fistula can be localized at different levels, the most frequent being the pulmonary and coronary fistulas (Figure 8.8). A special type of arteriovenous communication is the one that can be established between the aorta and the pulmonary artery in cases of an anomalous origin of the left coronary artery from the main pulmonary artery (Figure 8.9). In this anomaly, flow from the right coronary artery may drain into the pulmonary trunk through collateral arteries that connect both coronary arteries (right and left). If the shunt is important, it can cause myocardial ischemia due to a stealing phenomenon.

8.6 Atrial Septal Defect

Atrial septal defect (ASD) consists of a defect in the interatrial septum that permits communication between both atria. Four types of ASD can be distinguished: (1) *Ostium secundum*, the most frequent, the defect being placed in the middle of the interatrial septum, in the region of the fossa ovalis. (2) *Ostium primum*, where the defect is located in the most caudal part of the interatrial septum and it is associated with anomalies of the atrioventricular valves, usually a cleft in the left atrioventricular valve, causing valve regurgitation. (3) *Sinus venosus*, included among the atrioventricular ASD although it is located near the drainage of the venae cavae, most commonly placed in the cephalad part of the atrial septum, opposite the entry of the superior vena cava (superior vena cava defect), but sometimes being found posteriorly to posteroinferiorly to the fosa ovalis, near the entry of the inferior vena cava (inferior vena cava defect). In the superior vena cava type, an anomalous connection of right pulmonary veins, with a right superior pulmonary vein emptying directly into the right atrium or into the superior vena cava, is frequently associated. (4) Coronary sinus type ASD: it is an infrequent anomaly characterized by a defect in the coronary sinus roof, which permits communication between the left atrium and the right atrium through the coronary sinus[14].

The volume of the interatrial shunt, usually left-to-right, with the consequent right ventricle volume overload and increased pulmonary flow, depends on the size of the defect, but especially on the end-diastolic

F. 8.5. (A) Spin echo image, axial plane, showing a persistent left superior vena cava. (B) Image in spin echo, coronal plane, showing in a longitudinal section (arrow) a persistent left superior vena cava draining into the coronary sinus. AAo: ascending aorta; Ao: aorta; CS: coronary sinus; DAo: descending aorta; LSVC: left superior vena cava; MPA: main pulmonary artery; RA: right atrium; RPA: right pulmonary artery; RSVC: right superior vena cava; Tr: trachea.

F. 8.6. Coronal section with gradient echo technique that shows an anomalous right pulmonary venous drainage at the level of the junction between inferior vena cava and right atrium (arrow), in a patient with scimitar's syndrome. A left pulmonary vein is seen, draining into the left atrium. Ao: aorta; LA: left atrium; PV: pulmonary vein; RA: right atrium; SVC: superior vena cava.

F. 8.7. The same patient as Figure 8.3. Spin echo axial slice showing the aorta situated anteriorly and to the right of an aneurysmatic pulmonary arterial trunk, which may be easily identified by its early bifurcation. This relationship of the great arteries is known as D-transposition. AAo: ascending aorta; LPA: left pulmonary artery; MPA: main pulmonary artery; RPA. right pulmonary artery.

114

FIGURE 8.8A and B

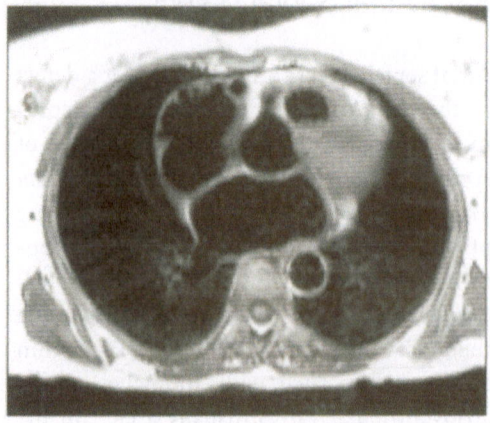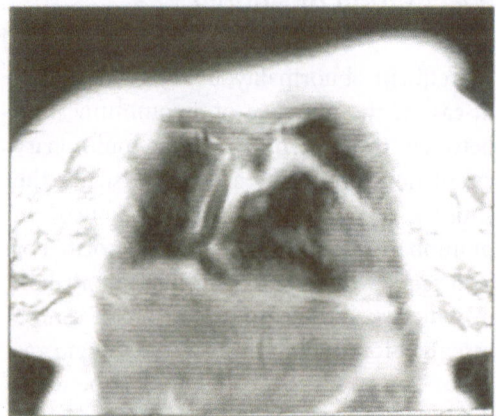

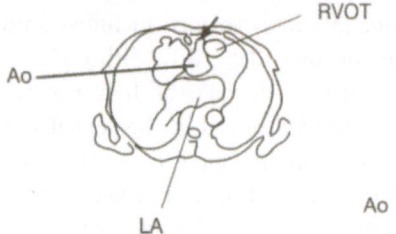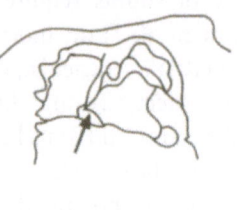

FIGURE 8.9

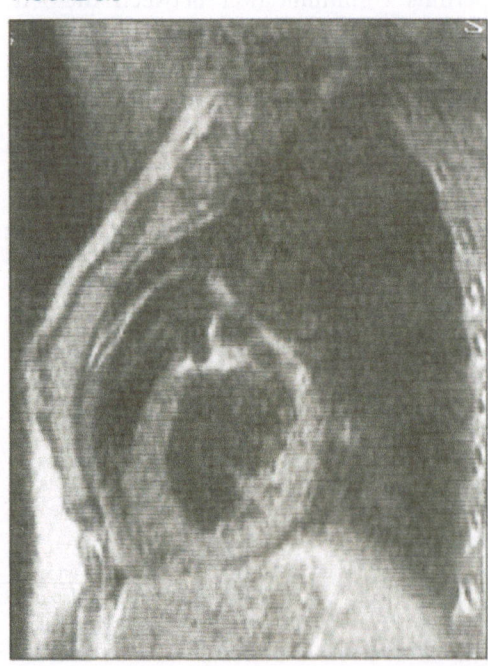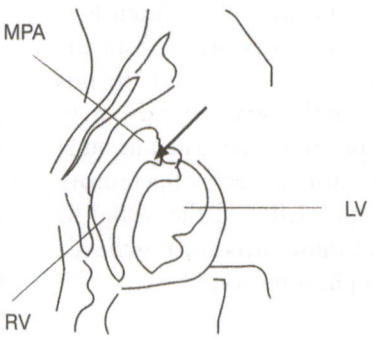

F. 8.8. Patient with a right coronary fistula draining into the coronary sinus. (A) Axial slice showing a right coronary artery very dilated in its proximal segment, with an anomalous origin and course, directed towards the anterior wall chest (arrow). (B) Coronal plane in a very anterior slice displaying a segment of the coronary artery fistula (arrow). Ao: aorta; LA: left atrium; RVOT: right ventricular outflow tract.

F. 8.9. Sagittal plane in spin echo technique showing the origin of the left coronary artery (arrow) from the posterior wall of the main pulmonary artery in a case of "anomalous origin of left coronary artery". LV: left ventricle; MPA: main pulmonary artery; RV: right ventricle.

ventricular pressure of both ventricles or, in other words, on the different compliance of both ventricular chambers.

MRI permits an easy evaluation of the size of the right cardiac chambers as well as the pulmonary arterial trunk and its main branches, giving indirect information about the volume of the shunt. Regarding the detection of the atrial septal defect, MRI is useful in the *ostium primum* type and, especially, in the *sinus venosus* type, where transthoracic echocardiography may have diagnostic problems, particularly in adult patients. In these cases, in contrast, MRI usually depicts the defect and also a frequently associated partial anomalous pulmonary venous connection to the superior vena cava (Figure 8.10 and 8.11). In *ostium secundum* ASD, MRI may produce eventual false-positive results due to the thinning of the fossa ovalis membrane; therefore, in this cases, special care should be taken and the atrial septum should be examined in various planes using, basically, axial slices[15]. The visualization of flow through the defect, by cine MR, will help to confirm the diagnosis. Velocity-encoded cine MRI may be used to quantify stroke flow in the aorta and main pulmonary artery,[16] and to estimate the shunt volume, by calculating the relation of flows (Qp:Qs)[17].

8.7 Ventricular Septal Defect

Ventricular septal defect (VSD) consists of an orifice in the interventricular septum. It may be small or large, restrictive or nonrestrictive to blood flow, single or multiple, and may be placed in different regions. The VSD is classified as: a) muscular, when the edges of the defect are totally composed of muscular tissue; b) perimembranous, when they are located around the membranous septum and the central fibrous body constitutes one of its edges; c) subarterial, when it is situated below the pulmonary and aortic valves and there is aortopulmonary continuity. Muscular defects and perimembranous ones can be subclassified according to their location at the level of the inlet septum (near atrioventricular valves), the trabecular septum,

and/or the outlet septum. The volume of the shunt will be conditioned by the size of the VSD and the relationship between the pulmonary and the systemic vascular resistances. The progressive increase of the former will reduce the volume of the shunt, even leading to its inversion. It should be noted that, in some cases, the valvular structures surrounding the defect may progressively limit its size. For example, in subtricuspid defects, the growth of new fibrous tissue, coming from the tricuspid valve or from the membranous septum, may seal the defect. Likewise, in subaortic or subarterial perimembranous defects, the prolapse of the valve may progresively reduce the volume of the shunt ultimately closing the defect, but resulting in the development of aortic or pulmonary insufficiency, which in some cases can become severe and require a valvular prosthesis.

By using both axial longitudinal planes aligned with the interventricular septum (Figure 8.12), spin echo MRI technique may be used to visualize VSDs of moderate and large size[18], but because of its resolution it is not useful in the study of small VSDs[19], specially the muscular ones. Defects in the trabecular portion can be visualized from any view: axial, coronal or sagittal. It is important to complete the morphological study of the VSD with cine MRI using gradient-echo technique, because it will show the blood flow passing through the defect. When the defects are small, they may be diagnosed by visualization during systole of a signal loss in the right side of the interventricular septum, produced by the high velocity of the transorificial flow. Certainly, moving blood gives a high signal in cine MR, but in areas of turbulence the signal is lost. The outflow tract of the right ventricle should be analyzed systematically to diagnose a possible infundibular or valvular pulmonary stenosis associated with the ventricular septal defect.

8.8 Atrioventricular Defects

These occur as a consequence of an anomalous development of the endocardial cushions, which causes a defect in the atrioventricular

116

FIGURE 8.10A and B

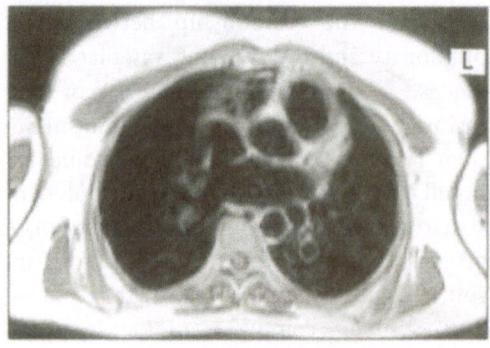

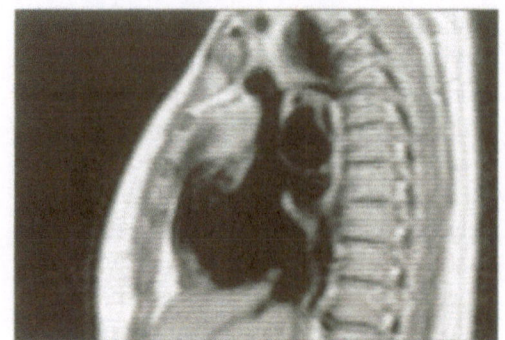

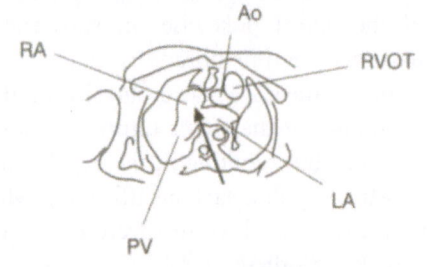

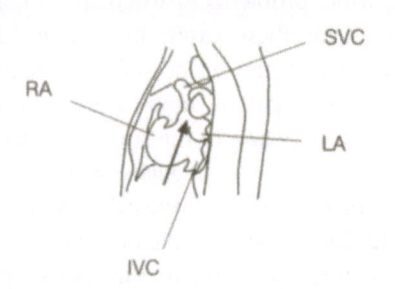

FIGURE 8.11

FIGURE 8.12

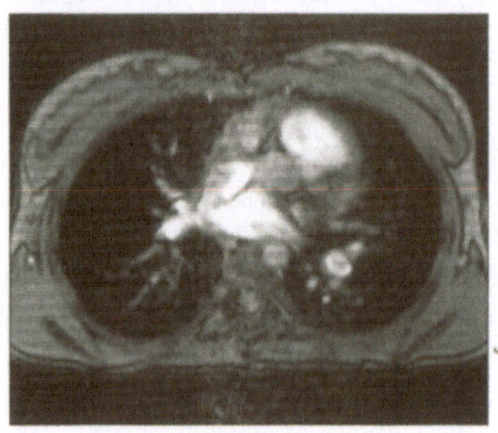

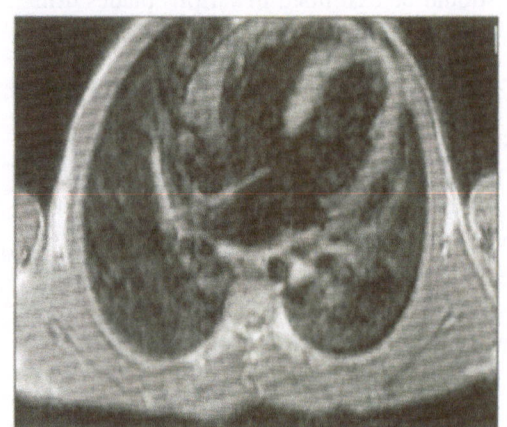

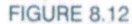

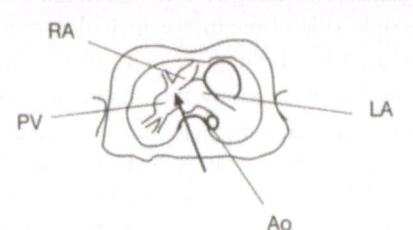

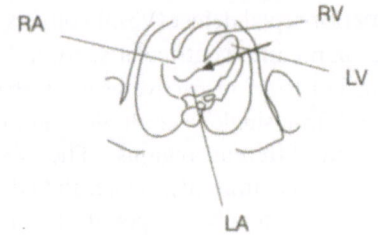

F. 8.10. Patient with a sinus venosus atrial septal defect, at the level of the entry of the superior vena cava. (A) axial slice and (B) sagittal slice. A defect in the high portion of the interatrial septum (arrows) can be seen in both images. Ao: aorta; IVC: inferior vena cava; LA: left atrium; PV: pulmonary vein; RA: right atrium; RVOT: right ventricular outflow tract; SVC: superior vena cava.

F. 8.11. Image in gradient echo of a sinus venosus atrial septal defect proximal to the entry of the superior vena cava showing a pulmonary vein (arrow) straddling the defect and draining into the right atrium. Ao: aorta; LA: left atrium; PV: pulmonary vein; RA: right atrium (vena cava/atrial junction).

F. 8.12. Four-chamber spin echo plane showing a perimembranous ventricular septal defect at the inlet portion of the ventricular septum (arrow). LA: left atrium; LV: left ventricle; RA: right atrium; RV: right ventricle.

septum as well as anomalies in the atrioventricular valves. There are partial forms, as it is the *ostium primum* ASD, characterized by the absence of the inferior or caudal portion of the atrial septum and a "cleft" at level of the left atrioventricular valve, causing regurgitation, and complete forms, made up of an atrial septal defect type *ostium primum* which extends down into the ventricular septum, and a single atrioventricular valve (complete atrioventricular canal). Between these two types, there are intermediate forms. All types of atrioventricular defects share the absence of the atrioventricular septum, both atrio-ventricular valves lying at the same level.

Using spin echo MRI to study the four chambers with axial planes (usually with slight obliquity), the absence of the typical unequal insertion of the atrioventricular valves into the interventricular septum as well as the septal defects can be observed[20]. Nevertheless, in the majority of patients, this information can be obtained by echocardiography. Therefore, MRI should be reserved for specific cases where diagnostic doubts persist, for example, to evaluate a possible small ventricular septal defect associated with an atrial septal defect with a single atrioventricular valve. In the last case, coronal slices with a slight obliquity can help in the diagnosis. Likewise, as MRI provides a wide view of all thoracic structures, it is a good technique to evaluate the size of heart chambers, allowing the detection of a possible disproportion of sizes among them, mainly between both ventricles, with dominance of either the morphologically left or right ventricle. This is especially important when a surgical correction is being evaluated, as the risk is higher and the results usually worse in cases with ventricular hypoplasia. Cine MRI may be useful to evaluate valve function. Sometimes it may give more information than echocardiography about blood jet direction and its consequences. For example, in cases of *ostium primum* atrial septal defect, the left atrioventricular valve regurgitation may be directed toward the right atrium throught the atrial septal defect. There is a mandatory shunt from the left ventricle to the right atrium, which may be responsible for early clinical symptoms.

8.9 Patent Ductus Arteriosus

The ductus arteriosus, the most common type of extracardiac shunt, represents persistent patency of the vessel that in the fetus normally connects the pulmonary artery and the aorta, 5–10 mm below the origin of the left subclavian artery. Usually, it closes after birth, first by contraction of the medial smooth muscle (functional closure) and later by connective tissue formation and fibrosis. By 2–3 weeks the closure is completed. If the vessel remains open, a shunt results, normally left-to-right, from the aorta to the pulmonary artery. This anomaly is called patent or persistent ductus arteriosus (PDA). If the increased pulmonary flow is significant, a dilatation of the left chambers and the ascending aorta will result. Children with a large PDA may show a progressive elevation in pulmonary vascular resistence, as a consequence of the development of a pulmonary vasculopathy, eventually resulting in reversal of the shunt and differential cyanosis (cyanosis in the inferior limbs with a more rose-colored coloration in the superior limbs, corresponding to Eisenmenger's syndrome).

In small children, PDA can be usually diagnosed by 2D-Doppler echocardiography, but this may be difficult in adult patients. It is in these cases where MRI can be useful[21], using the spin echo technique and in coronal or sagittal planes with a slight obliquity (Figure 8.13), or, even better, using cine MRI. If the ductus is small, short or tortuous, MRI can give rise to a false-negative result.

8.10 Obstructive Lesions

Valvular stenosis is discussed in another section of this book (Chapter 4), the basic concepts explained there being also applicable to congenital valvular stenosis.[22] This section will be specifically dedicated to the study of: 1) right ventricular outflow obstruction, 2) valvular and supravalvular pulmonary stenosis, 3) fixed subvalvular and supravalvular aortic stenosis, and 4) coarctation of the aorta.

a. Right ventricular outflow tract obstruction

MRI is very useful for the morphological analysis of the myocardium. It can easily visualize a hypertrophied right ventricle helping also in identifying the distribution of hypertrophy: i.e.: diffuse, shaped by ventricular bands, or located at the infundibular level, with the consequent obstruction to ventricular ejection[23] (see the section devoted to Tetralogy of Fallot). The measurement of blood velocity by phase mapping techniques permits calculation of the gradient, as may be accomplished by conventional Doppler techniques. Infundibular obstruction will be better observed in coronal planes or in those oblique planes that can be aligned longitudinally with the right ventricular outflow tract.

b. Valvular and supravalvular pulmonary stenosis

Pulmonary valve morphology is not easily assessed using MRI. Only thickened and dysplastic valves with restricted opening can be visualized with MR, especially using the spin echo technique. It is easier to detect a hypertrophied right ventricle, with a possible associated infundibular obstruction, as well as a poststenotic dilated pulmonary arterial trunk[24]. By means of the typical image of signal void, the gradient echo technique permits visualization of a turbulent flow at valvular or subvalvular level. If velocity phase mapping is available, the valvular or subvalvular pulmonary gradient can be calculated.

Supravalvular stenosis, generally ring-shaped, can be located above the valve, at the level of the pulmonary arterial trunk, which shows an hour-glass shaped morphology, or at the level of the distal pulmonary branches, which are usually multiple. In the latter cases, their visualization by MRI can be difficult, and for diagnosis it may be necessary to look for the narrowing of the flow signal or the signal loss using the gradient echo technique.

c. Subvalvular and supravalvular aortic stenosis

Dynamic obstruction of the left ventricular outflow was discussed in the section dealing with cardiomyopathies; therefore, only subvalvular fixed stenosis will be studied here. These can consist of a fibrous or fibromuscular ring, or may be more diffuse, presenting with a true tunnel throughout the outflow tract. These anomalies are usually diagnosed by echocardiography. Nevertheless, in cases with a difficult echocardiographic window, MRI spin echo technique using oblique slices similar to the left anterior oblique projection in angiography can be useful to study subaortic morphology. At the same time it provides information about the degree of secondary hypertrophy of the left ventricle. The gradient echo technique will confirm the level of obstruction, and the flow analysis by velocity mapping will permit calculation of the gradient.

Supravalvular stenosis, normally consisting of a fibrous ring near the aortic valve, is much less frequent. In contrast to aortic subvalvular stenosis, MRI plays an important role in its study. It can provide morphological information by means of the spin echo technique and functional information by means of velocity mapping.

d. Coarctation of the aorta

Coarctation of the aorta consists of a constriction of the aortic lumen, usually discrete, sometimes of significant length, generally located at the beginning of the descending aorta, after the origin of the left subclavian artery, but in rare cases placed at level of aortic arch or even at abdominal aorta. Mainly in older children, adolescents and adults, large collateral vessels develop from the subclavian artery and its branches to intercostal arteries below the coarctation to give the classic appearance of rib notching on the chest roentgenogram.

As occurs with other anomalies of the aortic arch, MRI is the noninvasive preferred technique to demonstrate and evaluate before surgery a patient with suspected coarctation of the aorta[25] (Figure 8.14 and 8.15), specially in the older child, adolescent or adult, as Doppler echocardiography may not adequately display the lesion. MRI in spin echo or gradient echo (cine MRI) techniques may locate the lesion, show its morphology, length and severity (Figure 8.16), the size of the aortic isthmus and the aorta at the pre- and post-coarctation levels, and possible large collateral vessels (Figure 8.17). In summary,

FIGURE 8.13

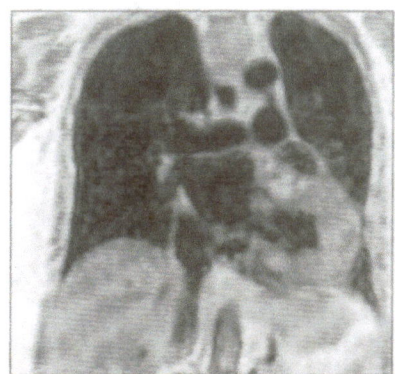

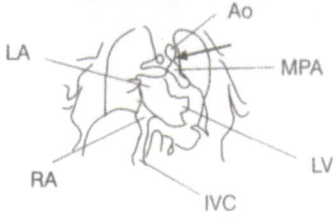

FIGURE 8.14

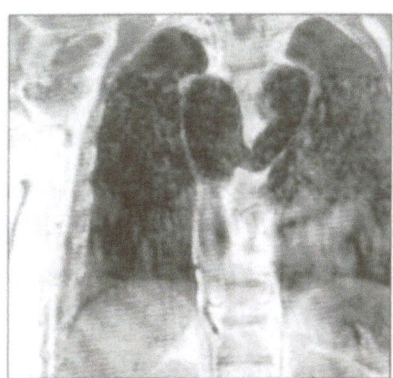

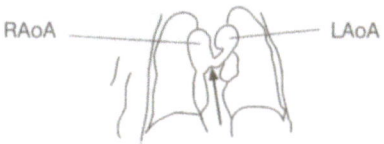

FIGURE 8.15

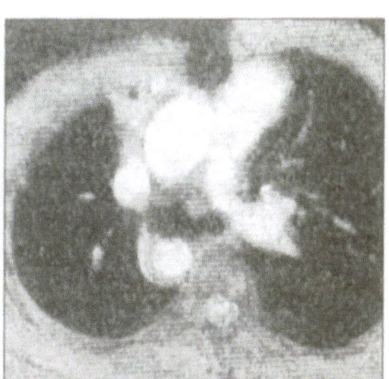

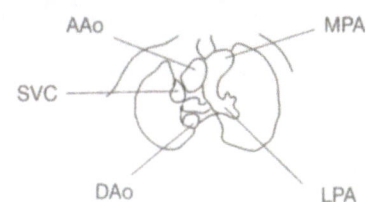

FIGURE 8.16A and B

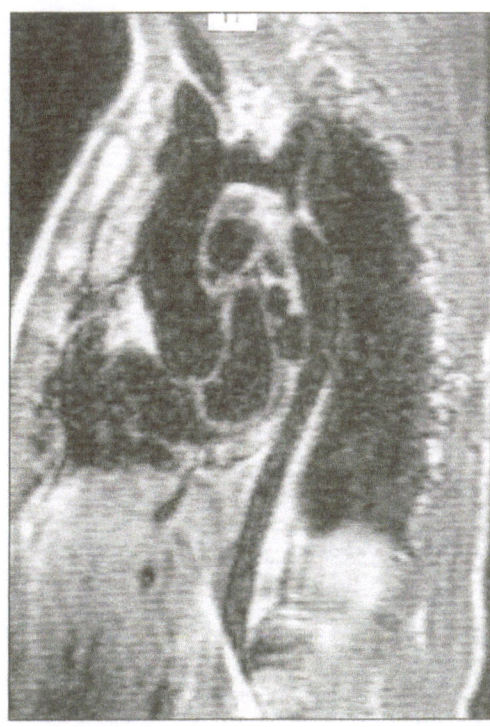

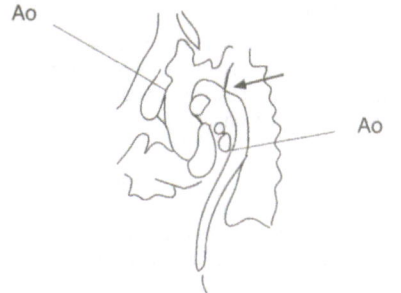

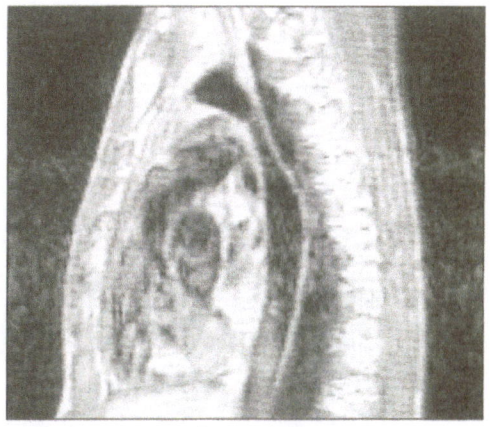

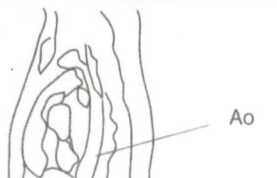

F. 8.13. Coronal plane showing the presence of a patent ductus arteriosus (arrow) connecting the aorta and the main pulmonary artery. Ao: aorta; IVC: inferior vena cava; LA: left atrium; LV: left ventricle; MPA: main pulmonary artery; RA: right atrium.

F. 8.14. Double aortic arch. Spin echo coronal plane, showing the left and right aortic archs and their union (arrow) to form a single descending aorta. LAoA: left aortic arch; RAoA: right aortic arch.

F. 8.15. Axial slice in gradient echo showing the descending aorta to the right of the rachis in a case of right aortic arch. Furthermore, there is agenesis of the right pulmonary artery. AAo: ascending aorta; DAo: descending aorta; LPA: left pulmonary artery; MPA: main pulmonary artery; SVC: superior vena cava.

F. 8.16. Coarctation of the aorta. (A) Oblique sagittal plane showing a typical discrete coarctation of the aorta located (arrow) below the origin of the left subclavian artery. (B) Sagittal plane displaying a long tubular aortic coarctation. Ao: aorta.

FIGURE 8.17

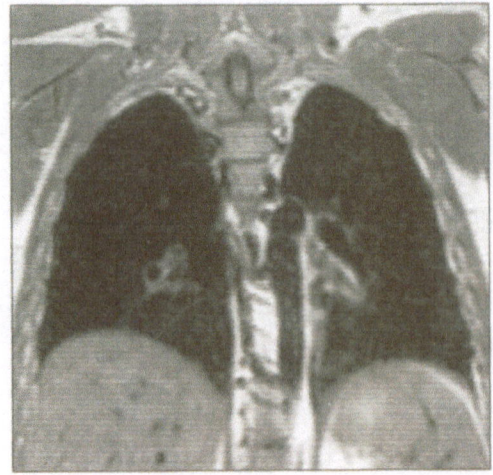

FIGURE 8.18

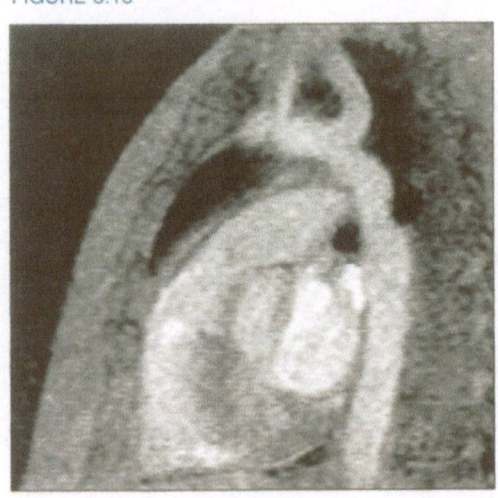

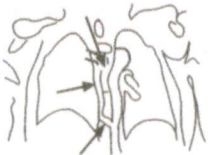

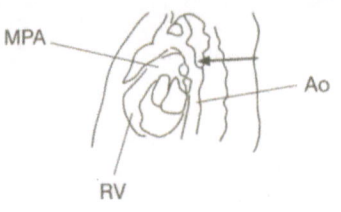

FIGURE 8.19

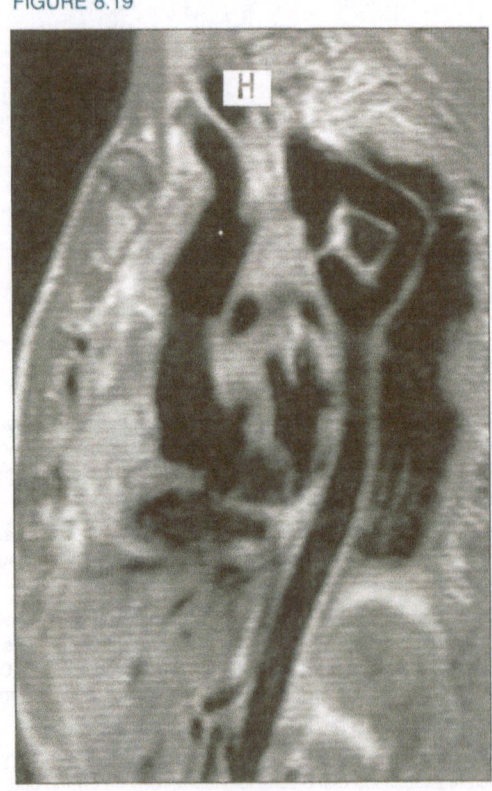

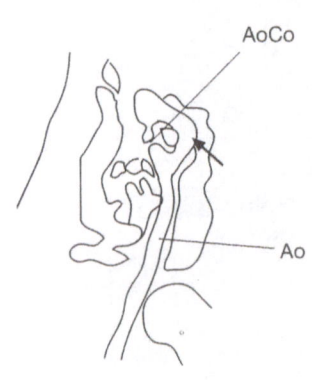

F. 8.17. Coronal plane spin echo image of a patient with coarctation of the aorta. Large collateral vessels may be seen (arrows).

F. 8.18. Saggital plane gradient echo after surgical correction of an aortic coarctation. A patch was used to repair the stenotic lesion (arrow). Ao: aorta; MPA: main pulmonary artery; RV: right ventricle.

F. 8.19. Spin echo image after surgery for aortic coarctation: A prosthetic conduit from the aorta, above the coarctation, to the descending aorta, below the coarctation, was used. Note the 90º angle twisting of the conduit, but without evidence of obstruction into it. Ao: aorta; AoCo: aortic coarctation.

together with the external gradient (difference in systolic arterial pressure between the superior and inferior limbs), it provides all the necessary information prior to surgery.[26]

The best planes are usually the axial and oblique ones, specifically the oblique left anterior. Attempts must be always made to obtain a slice aligned longitudinally with the coarctated area. Incorrect alignments can give rise to false positives or to exaggerate the severity of the obstruction.

As a consequence of its high anatomical resolution, MRI is also the best technique to evaluate the surgical results, independently of the type of surgery (end-to-end anastomosis, patch, tubular graft, etc.) (Figures 8.18 and 8.19), or the results of balloon catheter angioplasty. It also permits detection of possible complications related to the therapeutic procedure used (aortic aneurysm, aortic dissection, periaortic hematoma).

8.11   Complex Congenital Heart Diseases

Complex congenital heart lesions refer to anomalies characterized by the association of various defects. Some associations may be even necessary for the development to term of the fetus. In order to consider eventual surgery and/or to make a prognosis, it is nesessary to identify all of the lesions. MRI usually provides important morphological and functional information, but in order to complete the study, it is used in combination with Doppler echocardiography and frequently with conventional cardiac catheterization. Some of these anomalies will be described in the next paragraphs.

a. Tetralogy of Fallot

Fallot's Tetralogy is the most frequent cyanotic congenital heart disease, especially in patients over two years of age. It basically consists of: a) extensive subaortic ventricular septal defect; b) dextroposition of the aorta origin; c) infundibular pulmonary stenosis; d) right ventricular hypertrophy. Other frequently associated anomalies are: valvular pulmonary stenosis, stenosis of the pulmonary branches, right aortic arch, atrial septal defect, anomalies in the origin and course of the coronary arteries, etc. The treatment of this anomaly requires surgery, either palliative or corrective. The shunting operations (palliative) increase pulmonary flow, but they should be regarded as preliminary to more complete correction. The more usual surgical shunt is the Blalock-Taussig fistula, which connects the subclavian artery with the pulmonary artery. Anatomical correction consists of closing the ventricular septal defect by a patch, and relieving the infundibular stenosis by excision of the obstructing muscle bundles. In cases of associated pulmonary valve stenosis, it will be necessary to perform a pulmonary valvotomy. If relief of the obstruction remains incomplete, an outflow patch may be incorporated into the ventriculotomy closure, enlarging the ventricular outflow. When the pulmoanry annulus and the main pulmonary artery are small, the patch may be extended from the infundibulum to the pulmonary artery trunk, but that may cause an important pulmonary regurgitation. MRI can be useful for the study of the Tetralogy of Fallot, providing additional information to that rendered by Doppler echocardiography.[27] Apart from those cases with a poor echocardiographic window, the basic lesions can be easily visualized by using either one of both techniques (Figure 8.20A), but MRI has proved to be superior to echocardiography in evaluating the size of the pulmonary arterial trunk and its branches (Figure 8.20B), its growth following palliative surgery (important data when posterior corrective surgery is under consideration), the existence of possible supravalvular pulmonary stenosis, etc. Nevertheless, both techniques have limitations in the study of the origin and course of the coronary arteries, which make the use of cardiac catheterization necessary before corrective surgery.

To study Fallot's Tetralogy by MRI, sections in various planes should be made: axial, sagittal, coronal, sometimes with slight obliquity. For example, transverse slices with ascending obliquity in an antero-posterior projection (similar to the sitting-up plane in angiography) are extremely useful to study the pulmonary arterial trunk and its main branches. By gradient echo MRI it is easy to diagnose whether these branches are hypoplastic, since it allows them to be distinguished from the adjacent bronchi. As a general rule, the left pulmonary artery runs above the main left bronchus, which is posterior to the left pulmonary veins. On the right side, the main right bronchus is posterior to the right pulmonary artery, while the pulmonary veins are placed anteriorly and inferiorly. It should be noted that when a pulmonary artery is absent a gradient echo study also facilitates the diagnosis (Figure 8.15)

b. Truncus arteriosus

This consists of the presence of a single vessel straddling a ventricular septal defect and from which the aorta and the pulmonary artery arise. This vessel collects the blood from both ventricles. There are different varieties of truncus arteriosus, depending on the way in which the pulmonary arteries originate. The identification of these vessels is very important, both for the classification of the anomaly and for the evaluation of the possibilities and type of surgery.

Pulmonary atresia with ventricular septal defect was known in the past as type IV truncus. In this anomaly, pulmonary vascularization can be extraordinarily anomalous, with major aorto-pulmonary collaterals (MAPCA) coming off generally from the descending aorta below the isthmus and sometimes from the subclavian arteries, supplying different portions of the lungs. Pulmonary artery development varies from complete absence of all central pulmonary arteries, an absent trunk and one branch, and one absent branch to one side, to completely developed pulmonary arteries beyond an atretic but imperforate pulmonary valve.

The use of MRI can provide important anatomical information about any type of truncus [28] (Figures 8.21 and 8.22) as well as about pulmonary atresia with ventricular septal defect. It is necessary to evaluate different planes for the complete study of the pulmonary arteries, and especially of the aorto-pulmonary collaterals (Figure 8.23), the visualization of which is difficult, even using angiography.

c. Complete transposition of the great arteries

This anomaly is characterized by the association of atrioventricular concordance with ventriculoarterial discordance. The anatomical arrengement results in two separate and parallel circulations. Some communication between the two circulations is necessary for survival. The minimum communications which permit subsistence of the newborn are the foramen ovale and the ductus arteriosus, but they tend to close in the first few days of life, making it necessary to perform some paliative technique, such as a transcatheter balloon atrial septostomy, and/or a corrective operation.

In the most common type of complete transposition of the great arteries, the aortic valve (and the initial portion of the ascending aorta) is usually placed in front of and to the right of the pulmonary valve, a position which is known as D-transposition. The aorta and the pulmonary artery do not cross, but they rather run parallel. The most frequent associated anomalies are ventricular septal defect (30% of the cases) and pulmonary stenosis.

Although the diagnosis is usually accomplished by echocardiography in the first week of life, MRI can be very useful to study children or adult patients, after an atrial (venous) or an arterial switch operation and in order to evaluate some residual lesions and or sequelae of complications from the operation. Coronal planes usually allow good visualization of the ventriculoarterial connection, while sagittal planes display the antero-posterior relationship of the great vessels (Figures 8.24 and 8.25). The latter are especially useful in order to demonstrate the origin of the aorta from the right ventricle. Axial slices help in diagnosing the position of the arteries and in their identification. Associated anomalies, mainly ventricular septal defect or/and pulmonary stenosis may be demonstrated in axial and coronal planes. In patients undergoing physiological surgical correction (the systemic venous return is diverted into the left ventricle through the mitral valve, and then to the pulmonary artery, while the pulmonary venous return is diverted through the tricuspid valve to the right ventricle and the aorta), whether by the Mustard [29] or Senning [30] technique, MRI

FIGURE 8.20A and B

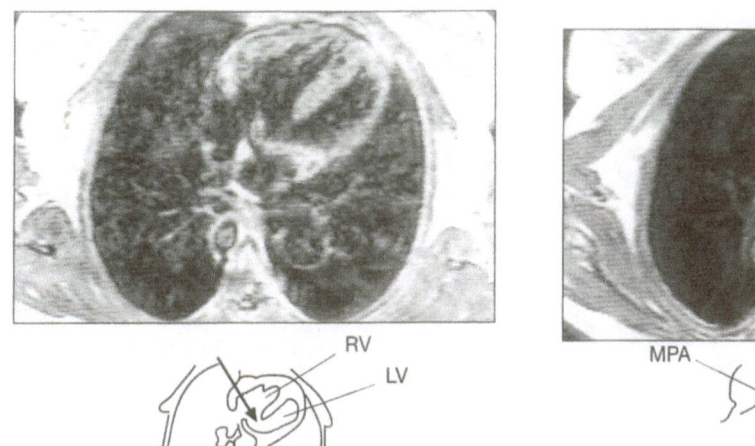

FIGURE 8.21A and B

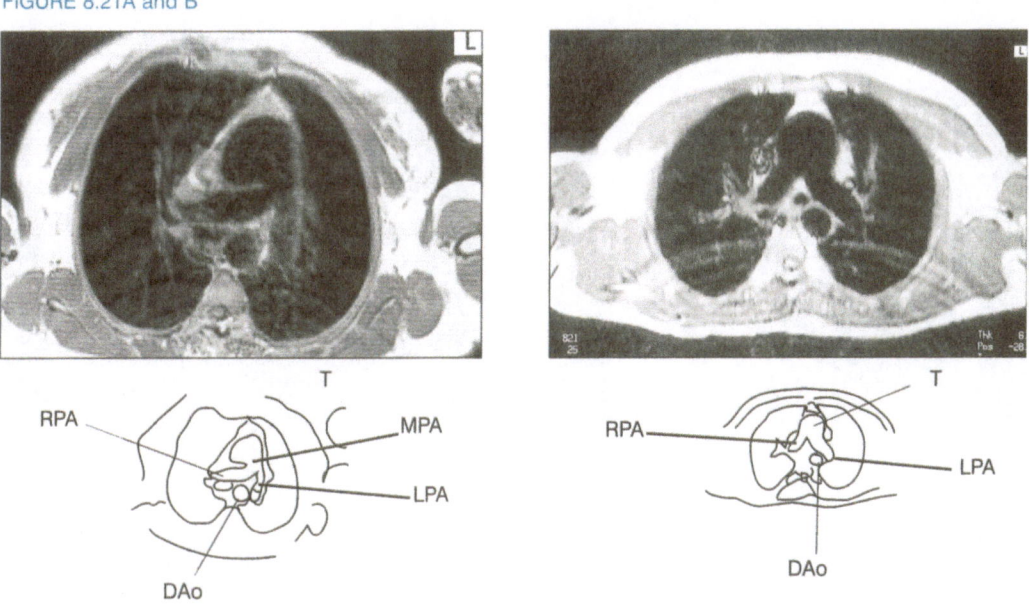

FIGURE 8.22A and B

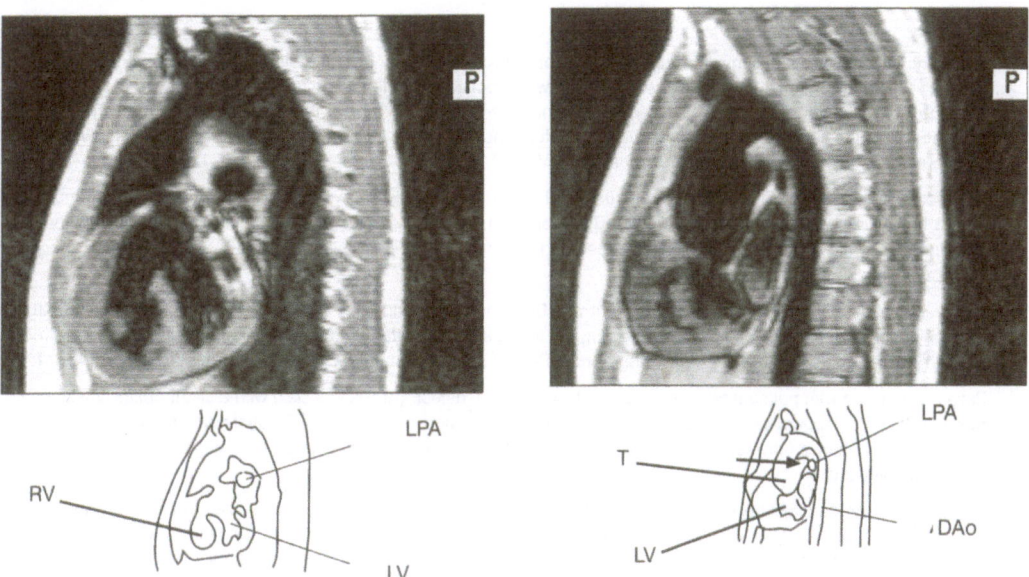

FIGURE 8.23A and B

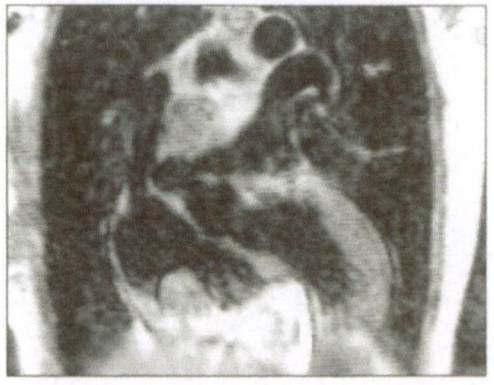

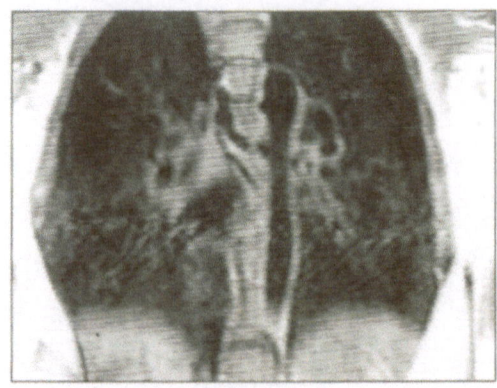

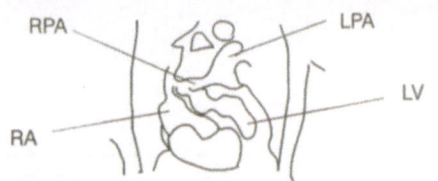

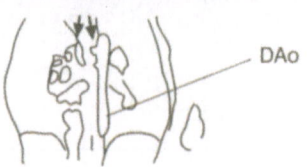

FIGURE 8.24A and B

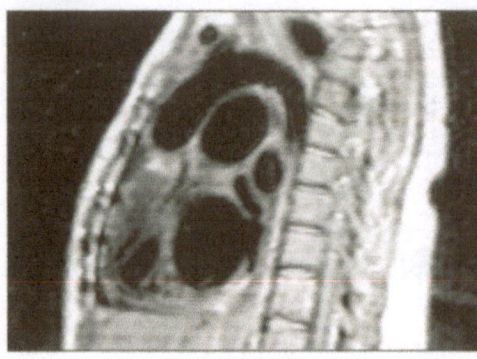

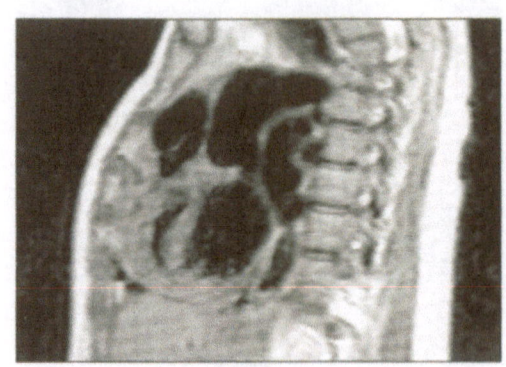

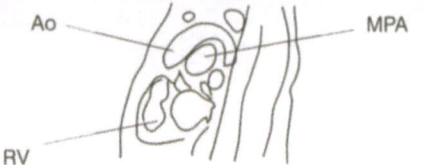

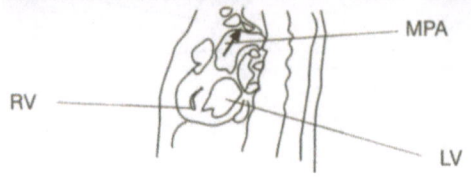

F. 8.20. Spin echo images from a patient with Tetralogy of Fallot. (A) Axial slice with a slight obliquity showing a ventricular septal defect in the upper part of the ventricular septum (arrow) associated with right ventricular hypertrophy. (B) Axial plane with slight obliquity (sitting-up position), displaying the infundibular obstruction (arrow) and the main pulmonary artery with its branches. Note the significant dilatation of the distal left pulmonary artery. LPA: left pulmonary artery; LV: left ventricle; MPA: main pulmonary artery; RPA: right pulmonary artery; RV: right ventricle.

F. 8.21. Spin echo sagittal slices. (A) Patient with truncus type I. See the main pulmonary artery arising from the large truncal vessel and its bifurcation into left and right branches. (B) Patient with truncus type II. Note that the left and right pulmonary arteries arise independently from the truncus. DAo: descending aorta; RPA: right pulmonary artery; LPA: left pulmonary artery; MPA: main pulmonary artery; T: truncus.

F. 8.22. Spin echo images of a type II truncus in a patient with Eisenmenger's syndrome. (A) Sagittal plane showing the subtruncal ventricular septal defect. (B) Sagittal slice showing the truncus and the left pulmonary artery originating posteriorly from the great truncal vessel (arrow). DAo: descending aorta; LPA: left pulmonary artery; LV: left ventricle; RV: right ventricle; T: truncus.

F. 8.23. Patient diagnosed with pulmonary atresia with ventricular septal defect. (A) Sagittal slice with a slight obliquity (sitting-up position) showing a pulmonary arterial trunk in continuity with its main branches. (B) Coronal plane showing the presence of aortic collateral arteries (arrows). DAo: descending aorta; LPA: left pulmonary artery; LV: left ventricle; RA: right atrium; RPA: right pulmonary artery.

F. 8.24. Patient with dextrocardia, situs inversus, atrioventricular concordance and ventriculoarterial discordance that was submitted to a Mustard operation. Sagittal slices at different levels showing the anterior position of the aorta in relation to the pulmonary arterial trunk. (A) The aorta can be identified by its elongated image which gives rise to the aortic arch. (B) The pulmonary artery bifurcates (arrow) into its two main branches. Ao: aorta; LV: left ventricle; MPA: main pulmonary artery; RV: right ventricle.

allows the study of a possible obstruction at level of the systemic or the pulmonary venous return, which is one of the most frequent complications in this type of surgical repair. The use in these patients of pulsed Doppler with MRI provides the greatest sensitivity and specificity for the detection of an obstruction in the drainage of the superior vena cava.[31] Likewise, using the spin echo, and cine-MRI, it is possible to study the right ventricular function and to calculate the ejection fraction, which is important data, as in these cases the right ventricle works as a systemic ventricle. In those patients who have been submitted to a Jatene type of anatomical correction[32] (arterial switch), MRI is useful to study the new ventriculoarterial connection (Figure 8.26), allowing diagnosis of a possible supravalvular stenosis at the level of the anastomosis and detection of possible valvular regurgitations, as well as a decreased ventricular function, by using cine MRI.

d. Tricuspid atresia

Tricuspid atresia is characterized by the absence of the right atrioventricular valve. It should be differentiated from cases with an imperforate tricuspid valve. In 65% of the cases, blood reaches the left atrium through a permeable foramen ovale, and in the remaining cases through an atrial septal defect. In the most common type, it is associated with atrioventricular and ventriculoarterial concordance, and the flow that reaches the left ventricle is diverted to the aorta and to the the right ventricle through a ventricular septal defect (called bulboventricular foramen, as tricuspid atresia is considered a type of single ventricle with absence of the right atrio-ventricular connexion). The size of the right ventricle and the pulmonary artery depends primarily on the pulmonary flow, which is related to the size of the bulboventricular foramen as well as the presence of an associated infudibular or valvular pulmonary stenosis, which occurs in approximately 15% of the cases. There are other types of tricuspid atresia, such as the one associated with ventriculoarterial discordance or the one which presents discordant atrioventricular connection and double outlet of the morphologically right ventricle, generally associated with juxtaposition of the

atrial appendages. The presence of pulmonary atresia with the aorta orginating from the single ventricle as a single vessel is less frequent. In the more typical form, a left ventricle of normal size or enlarged and a small-sized chamber corresponding to the right ventricle can be seen in axial planes using spin echo MR. The chamber is usually located in an anterior and right position, separated from the right atrium, which appears to be potentially connected to the left ventricle. This supports, as we have previously mentioned, the classification by some authors of this anomaly as a type of double atrioventricular inlet or single ventricle with atresia of the right atrioventricular valve. In the study of the atrioventricular connection, the absent valve is substituted by a dense and refringent band, in part composed of fat (sulcus tissue), making it necessary to take various slices to demonstrate that it extends to the center of the heart, and there is no tricuspid valve, and no hypoplastic one. A false-positive diagnosis of tricuspid atresia may be made if only an axial slice is evaluated, which may foreshorten the view of the right ventricle. MRI is also superior to echocardiography to evaluate potential candidates for surgical atrio-pulmonary connection (Fontan technique or similar) as it usually gives more complete information about the morphology and size of the pulmonary arteries, data which are very important, related with the prognosis.[33,34]

In patients who have undergone surgery, MRI with spin echo or gradient echo can be very useful to study the atriopulmonary connection[35]. It may help in the diagnosis of a possible obstruction at level of the connection, whether it has been accomplished directly (Figure 8.27) or with the interposition of prosthetic material[36]. Some authors have also shown that the technique of phase velocity mapping can be of help in this issue, since it provides information about velocity and volume of the pulmonary flow.[37]

e. Single ventricle

This corresponds to an anomaly in which both atrioventricular valves or a common atrioventricular valve open principally (more than 50%) into a single ventricular chamber. Another rudimentary ventricular cavity also exists that may have only a trabecular component, lacking the atrioventricular and ventriculoarterial connection, called a "trabeculated pouch", or may be composed of a trabecular component and an outlet tract with ventriculoarterial connection, when it is named the "outlet chamber." In any case, this rudimentary cavity does not have an atrioventricular inlet component, and, therefore, does not constitute a true ventricle. There are different types of single ventricle, depending on their morphology, their atrioventricular and their ventriculoarterial connections. Depending on their morphology they can be: (1) right-type single ventricle; (2) left-type single ventricle, or (3) indeterminate-type single ventricle, lacking a rudimentary chamber. They may have different types or modes of atrioventricular connection: by two valves, by a single valve; one of the valves may be absent; the valves can be hypoplastic or insufficient or they can be in a straddling or overriding position. Ventriculoarterial connection can also be of different types: concordant, discordant or "double outlet," etc., and pulmonary stenosis or atresia may exist. The most typical form consists of a left-type single ventricle with two atrioventricular valves and discordant ventriculoarterial connection. The outlet chamber is located in an anterior and usually left position, although it can be placed anteriorly and to the right or directly anterior. The aorta that arises from the outlet chamber is usually located in a position anterior and to the left of the pulmonary artery. When the ventriculoarterial connection is concordant, the pulmonary artery is situated anterior and to the left of the aorta. In some cases they can be placed side by side. In the right-type single ventricle, the rudimentary chamber is situated in a posterior position and, since the ventriculoarterial connection is usually of a "double outlet" type, it is normally small, composed only of the trabecular portion (trabeculated pouch). The double inlet atrioventricular connection, the presence of one or two atrioventricular valves (Figure 8.28), the morphology and trabeculation of the single ventricle, the position of the rudimentary chamber, the position of the interventricular septum and the presence, size and location of the bulboventricular foramen may be displayed by using the spin echo MRI technique with axial or four-chamber slices. This allows not only the diagnosis of the single ventricle but also classification and detection of some possible associated anomalies[38]. Sagittal (Figure 8.29) and coronal (Figure 8.30) slices are of great utility, especially for the study of the ventriculoarterial connection as well as for the localization of the great vessels. The gradient echo technique may confirm the diagnosis as it depicts the flow from both atria entering into a single ventricle cavity through the atrioventricular valvular floor. Likewise, it permits evaluation of the existence of possible valvular regurgitations.

f. Double outlet right ventricle

As the name suggests, in this type of anomaly, the two great vessels (aorta and pulmonary artery) arise from the right ventricle. Blood from the left ventricle drains into the right ventricle, through a ventricular septal defect. This orifice can be placed at subaortic, or subpulmonary position (Taussig-Bing), at the level of the inlet septum or separated from any valvular structure, at the level of the muscular septum, this point being important to consider with respect to surgical possibilities and results. The clinical manifestations basically depend on the size of the ventricular septal defect and on the presence or absence of an associated pulmonary stenosis. In cases of a large ventricular septal defect, without obstruction to the pulmonary flow, the symptoms are those of an important left-to-right shunt (except when it is associated with pulmonary arterial vasculopathy). When there is a significant pulmonary stenosis, the clinical picture mimics a case of Tetralogy of Fallot. The size of the ventricular septal defect is an important point. In cases of restrictive defects (muscular defects have a tendency to diminish in size) the blood flow from the systemic circuit and that from the pulmonary circuits will be obstructed.

As has been previously mentioned, the type of surgery and its results will basically depend on the relationship among the great vessels, the interventricular septal defect and the tricuspid valve, as well as on the associated anomalies, especially ventricular hypoplasia, ventricular cavities in a superior-inferior position, stenosis of pulmonary outflow tract or anomalies of the atrioventricular valves. MRI allows display of both great vessels arising from the right

FIGURE 8.25A and B

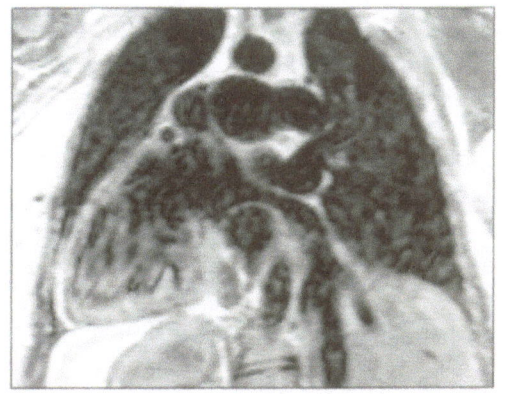

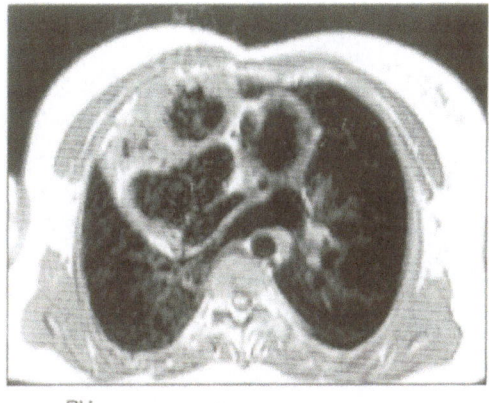

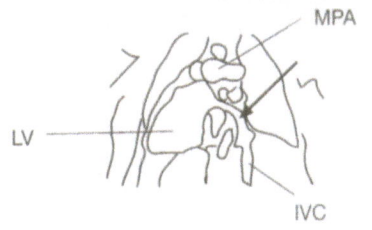

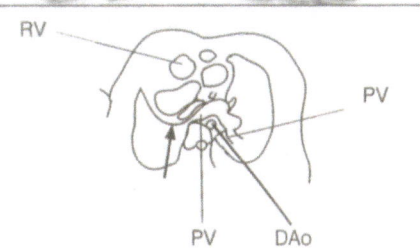

FIGURE 8.26A and B

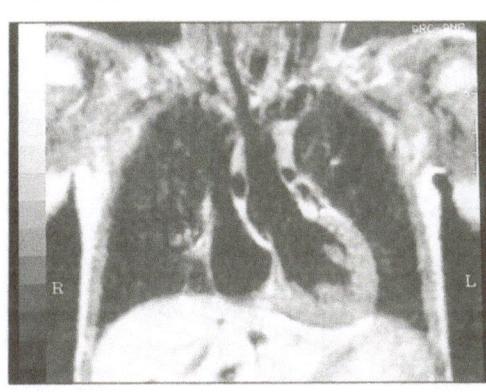

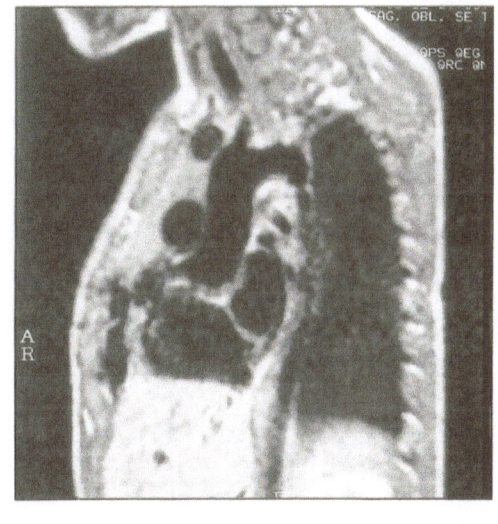

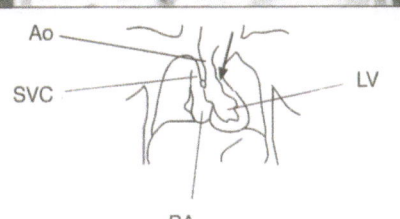

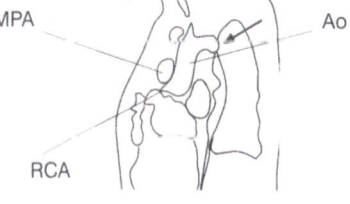

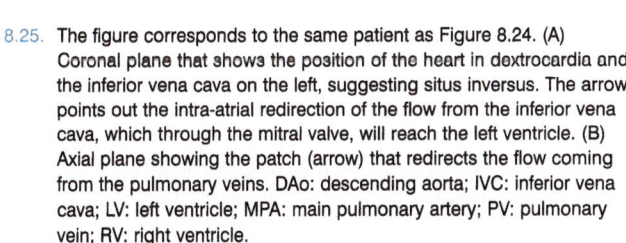

F. 8.25. The figure corresponds to the same patient as Figure 8.24. (A) Coronal plane that shows the position of the heart in dextrocardia and the inferior vena cava on the left, suggesting situs inversus. The arrow points out the intra-atrial redirection of the flow from the inferior vena cava, which through the mitral valve, will reach the left ventricle. (B) Axial plane showing the patch (arrow) that redirects the flow coming from the pulmonary veins. DAo: descending aorta; IVC: inferior vena cava; LV: left ventricle; MPA: main pulmonary artery; PV: pulmonary vein; RV: right ventricle.

F. 8.26. Jatene operation (arterial switch) in a patient with complete D-transposition of the great arteries (atrioventricular concordance with ventriculoarterial discordance). (A) Coronal spin echo plane showing the new emergence of the aorta from the morphologically left ventricle. Note the relatively abrupt reduction of the aorta at level of the anastomosis (arrow). (B) Oblique sagittal plane that shows the shape adopted by the aorta after being relocated in a position posterior to the pulmonary artery. An aortic coarctation can be observed at the beginning of the descending aorta (arrow). This lesion was not diagnosed prior to the surgical arterial switch, performed in the neonatal period. See the new origin of the right coronary artery, dilated and without stenosis at this level. Ao: aorta; LV: left ventricle; MPA: main pulmonary artery; RA: right atrium; RCA: right coronary artery; SVC: superior vena cava.

FIGURE 8.27

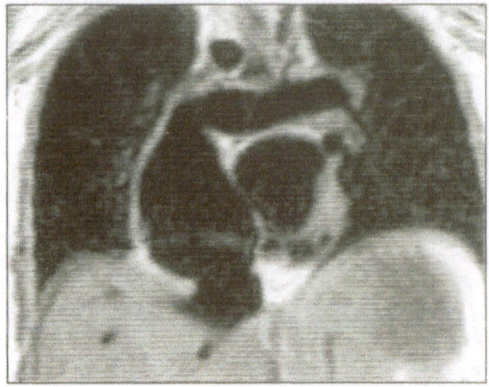

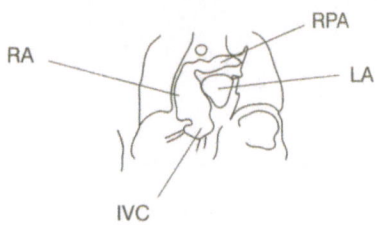

FIGURE 8.28

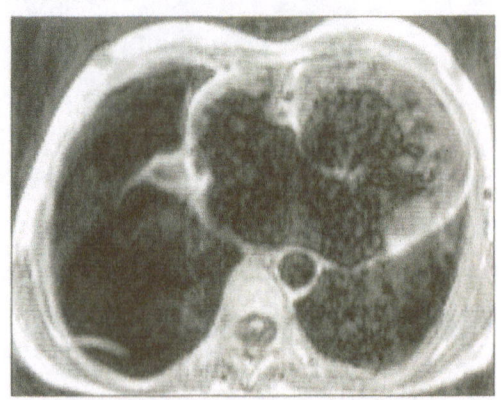

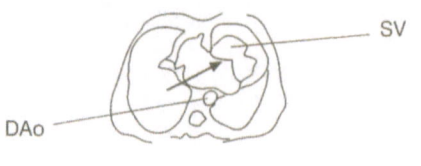

FIGURE 8.29A and B

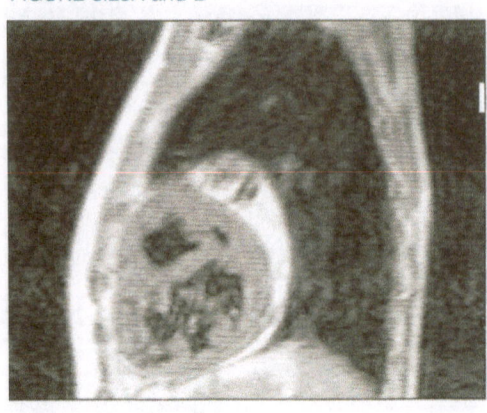

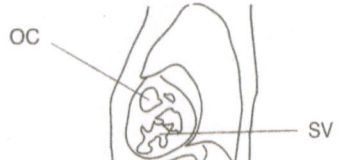

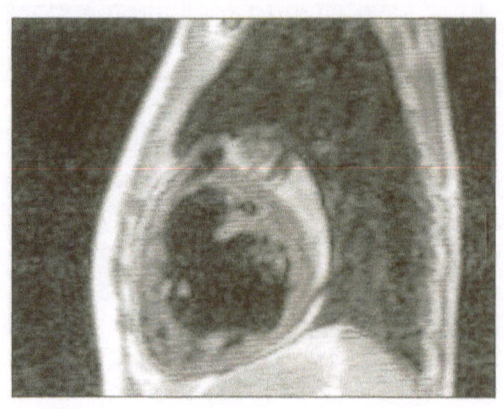

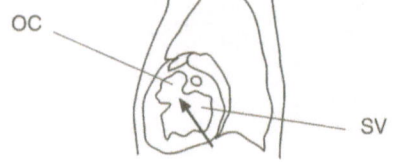

F. 8.27. Surgical atrio-pulmonary connection in a patient with complex congenital heart disease. Coronal plane, spin echo image showing the atriopulmonary connection between the roof of the right atrium and the pulmonary artery of the same side. IVC: inferior vena cava; LA: left atrium; RA: right atrium; RPA: right pulmonary artery.

F. 8.28. Axial plane that shows a single atrioventricular valve (arrow) in a case of double inlet left ventricular type. DAo: descending aorta; SV: single ventricle.

F. 8.29. Left type single ventricle. Sagittal planes from left (A) to right (B). Note the location of the outlet chamber in a superior position to the single ventricle. A large bulboventricular foramen (arrow) permits communication between both chambers. OC: outlet chamber; SV: single ventricle.

ventricle, and study of the morphology of the infundibular septum, by using axial slices at different levels and with the help of sagittal and coronal slices (occasionally with a certain obliquity), it permits localization and quantification of the size of the ventricular septal defect,[39] determination of the position and dimensions of the ventricular chambers, study of the outflow tracts and determination of the relative position of the great vessels. When the ventricular septal defect is subaortic, the aorta is usually in a position posterior and to the right (occasionally "side by side" and to the right) of the pulmonary artery. When the defect is subpulmonary, the aorta is usually in a position anterior and to the right of the pulmonary artery (Figures 8.31 and 8.32). Cine MRI can be helpful in the diagnosis of an associated pulmonary stenosis.

8.12   Postoperative Studies

Surgical treatment of congenital heart disease has greatly evolved during the last few years, and it has changed the survival rate of those patients suffering from complex congenital anomalies. A new population composed of adolescents or adults with complex congenital heart disease has emerged. A great number of these patients have been submitted to a type of surgery named "corrective", although rarely "curative". These patients usually present some residual lesions or sequelae from surgery, that require subsequent control. It is in these cases that MRI, without limitations concerning the acoustic window and with a wide field of vision, demonstrates its greatest utility. In this section we will concentrate on a few palliative techniques, such as surgical shunts and on pulmonary banding, since some corrective techniques have already been described in previous sections.

a. Surgical arteriovenous fistulas
The surgical performance of an arteriovenous shunt in order to increase pulmonary flow was the first surgical technique employed in patients with cyanotic congenital heart disease. Different types of fistulas exist, depending on the vessels used. The fistula of Blalock-Taussig consists of a termino-lateral anastomosis between the subclavian artery and the pulmonary artery on the same side. When this connection is made with the interposition of a prosthetic conduit, it is designated as "modified Blalock-Taussig fistula". Waterston and Potts fistulas are central shunts. In the former, the ascending aorta connects with the right pulmonary artery, while in the latter it is the descending aorta which connects with the left pulmonary artery. In both cases, the connection can be either direct or by means of prosthetic material. In the Glenn fistula, the right superior vena cava is connected to the right pulmonary artery . It may be done with (classic Glenn) or without disconnection of the right pulmonary artery from the pulmonary arterial trunk and the left pulmonary branch (Glenn bidirectional).

MRI is a highly useful technique for the morphological and functional study of surgical fistulas, due to its wide field of vision and its capacity for visualizing extracardiac structures.[40] In the majority of cases, it is necessary to analyze different projections and different section levels in order to carry out a complete study of the fistulas. Axial slices usually provide the necessary information for the study of Waterston and Potts fistulas, while sagittal and coronal slices are generally more useful for the study of Blalock-Taussig (Figure 8.33) and Glenn fistulas, which on occasion require a slight obliquity in order to obtain a better alignment of their course. By means of the spin echo technique and cine MRI it is possible to detect possible stenosis or distortions both of the fistula itself and of the pulmonary artery used in the anastomosis.

b. Banding of the pulmonary artery
In some types of congenital heart diseases with increased pulmonary flow, when corrective surgical treatment is not possible, the banding of the pulmonary arterial trunk with the purpose of decreasing the flow throughout the pulmonary circulation may be indicated. By using axial, sagittal and coronal slices, MRI may be useful to study it: it is even possible by using phase velocity mapping to calculate the gradient.[41] MRI is especially useful in those cases where the banding has migrated toward a superior portion of the pulmonary arterial trunk, and with a difficult visualization by echocardiography.

FIGURE 8.30A and B

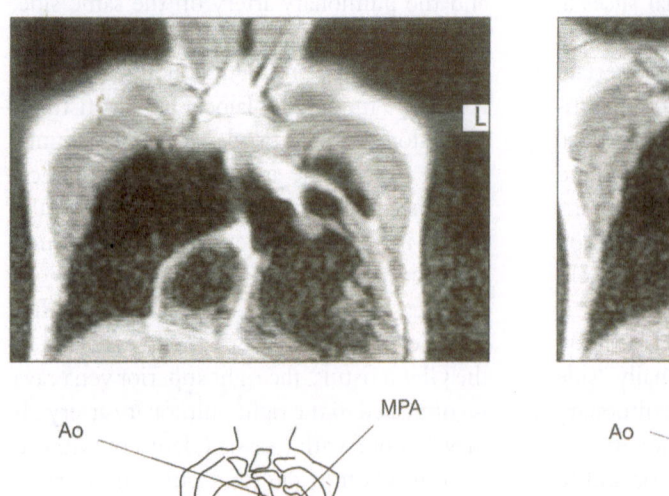

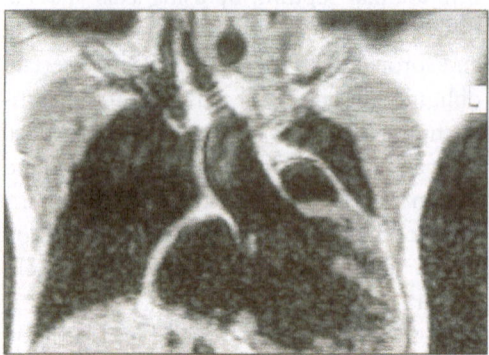

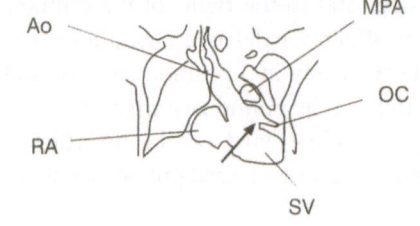

FIGURE 8.31A and B

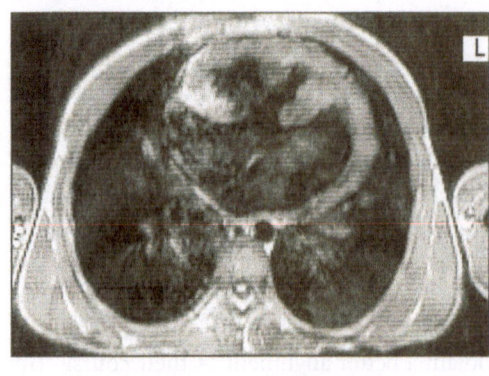

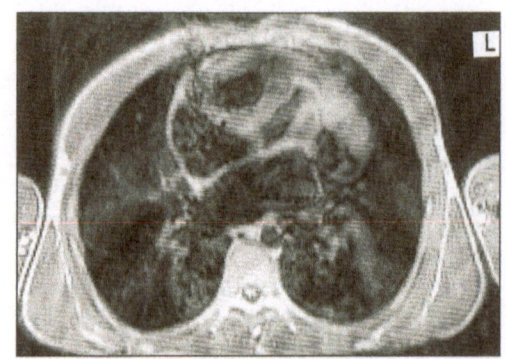

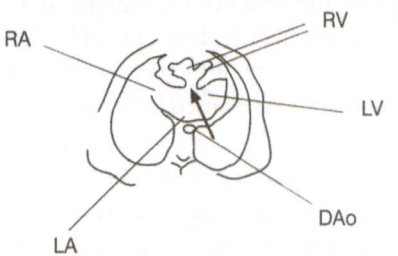

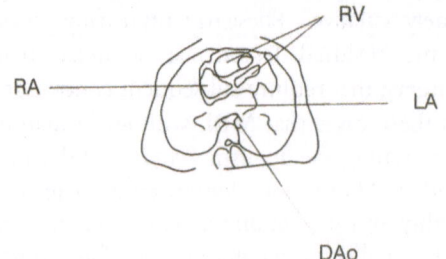

F. 8.30. Image corresponding to the same patient as in Figure 8.29. Coronal planes from anterior (A) to posterior (B). See the outlet chamber placed superior and to the left of the single ventricle. A large bulboventricular foramen links both chambers (arrow). The ventriculoarterial connection is concordant (aorta comes off the left type single ventricle, and pulmonary artery arises from the oulet chamber) and there is an associated infundibular pulmonary stenosis (arrowhead). Ao: aorta; MPA: main pulmonary artery; OC: outlet chamber; RA: right atrium; SV: single ventricle.

F. 8.31. Patient with double outlet right ventricle. Axial planes at different levels. (A) Inferior slice that shows the existence of a large perimembranous ventricular septal defect (arrow). (B) Superior slice where the double right ventricular outlet is displayed. DAo: descending aorta; LA: left atrium; LV: left ventricle; RA: right atrium; RV: right ventricle.

FIGURE 8.32A and B

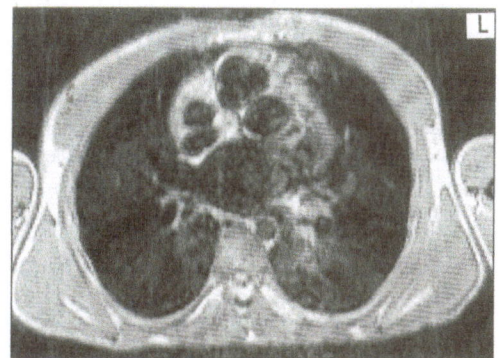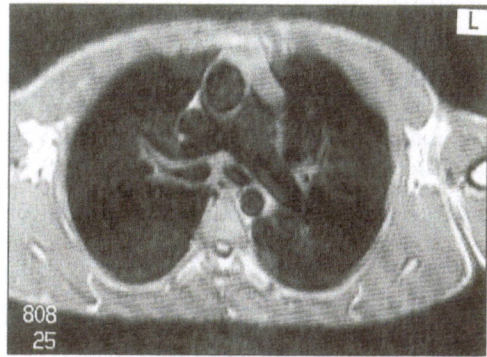

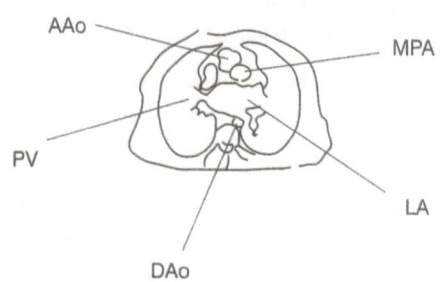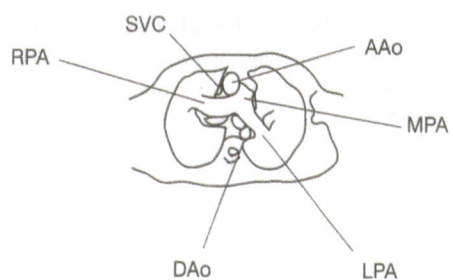

FIGURE 8.33

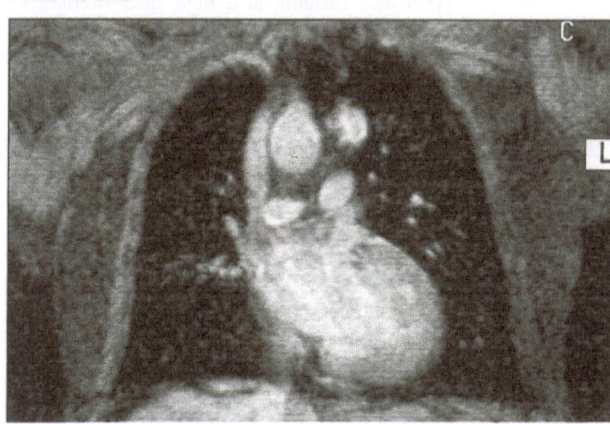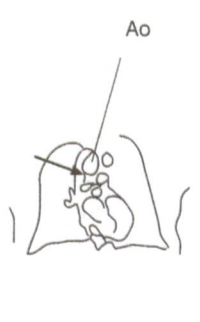

F. 8.32. The image corresponds to the same patient as in Figure 8.31. Axial slices are superior to those displayed in the previous figure. (A) Inferior plane showing both sigmoid valves at the same level. (B) Superior plane: the early bifurcation of the vessel placed on a left posterior position allows its identification as a pulmonary arterial trunk; the great vessels are in D-transposition. AAo: ascending aorta; DAo: descending aorta; LA: left atrium; LPA: left pulmonary artery; MPA: main pulmonary artery; PV: pulmonary vein; RPA: right pulmonary artery; SVC: superior vena cava.

F. 8.33. Coronal plane, gradient echo image, showing a functioning right Blalock-Taussig fistula (arrow). Ao: aorta.

References

1. Higgins ChB, Byrd BF, Farmer DW, Osaki L, Silverman NH, Cheitlin MD. Magnetic resonance imaging in patients with congenital heart disease. Circulation 1984; 70: 851–60.

2. Chung KJ, Simpson IA, Newman R. Sahn DJ, Sherman FS, Hesselink JR. Cine magnetic resonance imaging for evaluation of congenital heart disease: role in pediatric cardiology compared with echocardiography and angiography. J Pediatr 1988; 113: 1.028–1.035.

3. Simpson IA, Sahn DJ, Chung KJ. Noninvasive evaluation of congenital heart disease: Doppler ultrasound or magnetic resonance imaging. Echocardiography 1986; 6: 125–9.

4. Weinberg PM, Fogel MA. Cardiac MR imaging in congenital heart disease. Cardiol Clin 1998; 16: 315–48.

5. Hartnell GG, Cohen MC, Meier RA, Finn JP. Magnetic resonance angiography demonstration of congenital heart disease in adults. Clin Radiol 1996; 51: 851–7.

6. Hirsch R, Kilner PJ, Conelly MS, Redington AN, St John Sutton MG, Sommerville J. Diagnosis in adolescents and adults with congenital heart disease. Prospective assessment of individual and combined roles of magnetic resonance imaging and transesophageal echocardiography. Circulation 1994; 90: 2.937–2.951.

7. Boothroyd A. Magnetic resonance. Its current and future role in paediatric cardiac radiology. Eur J Radiol 1998; 26: 154–62.

8. Kersting-Sommerhoff BA, Diethelm L, Stanger P, et al. Evaluation of complex congenital ventricular anomalies with magnetic resonance imaging. Am Heart J 1990; 120: 133–42.

9. Masui T, Seelos KC, Kersting-Sommerhoff BA, Higgins ChB. Abnormalities of the pulmonary veins: evaluation with MR imaging and comparison with cardiac angiography and echocardiography. Radiology 1991; 181: 645–9.

10. Julsrud PR, Ehman RL. The "broken ring" sign in magnetic resonance imaging of partial anomalous pulmonary venous connection to the superior vena cava. Mayo Clin Proc 1985; 60: 874–9.

11. Wight CM, Barrat-Boyes BG, Calder AL, Neutze JM, Brandt PW. Total anomalous pulmonary venous connection: long-term results following repair in infancy. J Thorac Cardiovasc Sur 1977; 75: 52–63.

12. Katz NM, Kirklin JW, Pacifico AD. Concepts and practices in surgery for total anomalous pulmonary venous connection. Ann Thorac Surg 1978; 25: 479–87.

13. Gomes AS, Lois JF, Williams RG. Pulmonary arteries: MR imaging in patients with congenital obstruction of the right ventricular outflow tract. Radiology 1990; 174: 51–7.

14. Parsons JM, Baker EJ, Anderson RH, et al. Morphological evaluation of atrioventricular septal defects by magnetic resonance imaging. Br Heart J 1990; 64: 138–45.

15. Diethelm L, Dery R, Lipton MJ, Higgins CB. Atrial-level shunts: sensitivity and specificity of MR diagnosis. Radiology 1987; 162: 181–6.

16. Rees S, Firmin D, Mohiaddin R, Underwood R, Longmore D. Application of flow measurements by magnetic resonance velocity mapping to congenital heart disease. Am J Cardiol 1989; 64: 953–6.

17. Brenner LD, Caputo GR, Mostbeck G, et al. Quantification of left to right atrial shunts with velocity-encoded cine nuclear magnetic resonance imaging. J Am Coll Cardiol 1992; 20: 1.246–1.250.

18. Baker EJ, Ayton V, Smith MA, et al. Magnetic resonance imaging at a high field strength of ventricular septal defects in infants. Br Heart J 1989; 62: 305–10.

19. Didier D, Higgins CB. Identification and localization of ventricular septal defect by gated magnetic resonance imaging. Am J Cardiol 1986; 57: 1.363–1.368.

20. Wenink ACG, Ottenkamp J, Guit GL, Draulans Noe HA, Doornbos J. Correlation of morphology of the left ventricular outflow tract with two-dimensional Doppler echocardiography and magnetic resonance imaging in atrioventricular septal defect. Am J Cardiol 1989; 63: 1.137–1.140.

21. Chien CT, Lin CS, Hsu YH, Lin MC, Chen KS, Wu DJ. Potential diagnosis of hemodynamic abnormalities in patent ductus arteriosus by cine magnetic resonance imaging. Am Heart J 1991; 122: 1.065–1.072.

22. Kilner PJ, Firmin DN, O'Rees RS, et al. Valve and great vessels stenosis: assessment with MR jet velocity mapping. Radiology 1991; 178: 229–35.

23. Markiewicz W, Sechtem U, Higgins CB. Evaluation of the right ventricle by magnetic resonance imaging. Am Heart J 1987; 113: 8–14.

24. Wesley Vick III G, Rokey R, Huhta JC, Mulvagh SL, Johnston DL. Nuclear magnetic resonance imaging of the pulmonary arteries, subpulmonary region, and aortopulmonary shunts: a

comparative study with two-dimensional echocardiography and angiography. Am Heart J 1990; 119: 1.103–1.110.

25. Baker EJ, Ayton V, Smith MA, et al. Magnetic resonance imaging at high field strength of ventricular septal defects in infants. Br Heart J 1989; 62: 97–101.

26. Teien DE, Wendel H, Björnebrink J, Ekelund L. Evaluation of anatomical obstruction by Doppler echocardiography and magnetic resonance imaging in patients with coarctation of the aorta. Br Heart J 1993; 69: 352–5.

27. Mirowitz SA, Gutierrez FR, Canter CE, Vannier MW. Tetralogy of Fallot: MR imaging. Radiology 1989; 171: 207–12.

28. Sechtem U, Jungehülsing M, de Vivie R, Mennicken U, Höpp HW. Left hemitruncus in adulthood: diagnostic role of magnetic resonance imaging. Eur Heart J 1991; 12: 1.040–1.044.

29. Mustard WT. Successful two-stage correction of transposition of the great vessels. Surgery 1964; 55: 469–72.

30. Senning A. Surgical correction of transposition of the great vessels. Surgery 1959; 45: 966–9.

31. Campbell RM, Moreau GA, Johns JA, et al. Detection of caval obstruction by magnetic resonance imaging after intraatrial repair of transposition of the great arteries. Am J Cardiol 1987; 60: 688–91.

32. Jatene AD, Fontes VF, Souza LCB, Paulista PPA, Abdulmassih N, Soussa JEMR. Anatomic correction of transposition of the great arteries. J Thorac Cardiovasc Surg 1982; 83: 20–6.

33. Fogel MA, Donofrio MT, Ramaciotti C, Hubbard AM, Weinberg PM. Magnetic resonance and echocardiographic imaging of pulmonary artery size throught stages of Fontan reconstruction. Circulation 1994; 90: 2.927–2.936.

34. Julsrud PR, Ehmann RL, Hagler DJ, Ilstrup DM. Extracardiac vasculature is candidate for Fontan surgery: MR imaging. Radiology 1989; 173: 503–6.

35. Canter E, Gutierrez FR, Molina P, Hartmann AF, Spray TL. Noninvasive diagnosis of right-sided extracardiac conduit obstruction by combined magnetic resonance imaging and continuous-wave Doppler echocardiography. J Thorac Cardiovasc Surg 1991; 101: 724–31.

36. Donelly LF, Strife JL, Bailey WW. Extrinsic airway compresion secondary to pulmonary arterial conduits: MR findings. Pediatr Radiol 1997; 27: 268–70.

37. Rebergen SA, Ottenkamp J, Doornbos J, van der Wall EE, Chin JGJ, de Roos A. Postoperative pulmonary flow dynamics after Fontan surgery: assessment with nuclear magnetic resonance velocity mapping. J Am Coll Cardiol 1993; 21: 123–31.

38. Huggon IC, Baker EJ, Maisey MN, et al. Magnetic resonance imaging of hearts with atrioventricular valve atresia or double inlet ventricle. Br Heart J 1992; 68: 313–9.

39. Yoo SJ, Lim TH, Park IS, et al. MR anatomy of ventricular septal defect in double-outlet right ventricle with situs solitus and atrioventricular concordance. Radiology 1991; 181: 501–5.

40. Jacobstein MD, Fletcher BD, Nelson D, Clampitt M, Alfidi RJ, Riemenschneider TA. Magnetic resonance imaging: evaluation of palliative systemic-pulmonary artery shunts. Circulation 1984; 70: 650–6.

41. Simpson IA, Valdes-Cruz LM, Berthoty DP, et al. Cine magnetic resonance imaging and color Doppler flow mapping in infants and children with pulmonary artery bands. Am J Cardiol 1993; 71: 1.419–1.426.

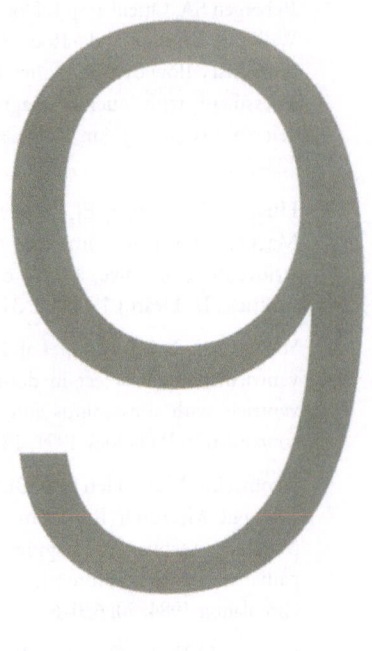

Contrast agents in cardiac MRI

G. PONS-LLADÓ

9.1 Introduction

In MRI studies, a contrast agent is defined as a substance that, once injected to the patient, modifies selectively the signal intensity of a particular anatomical structure by changing relaxation properties of tissues. Different magnetic substances have been tested, including manganese, gadolinium, dysprosium, and iron oxide, their effects depending on their pharmacokinetic properties and predominant action on proton relaxation.

Most contrast media used in MRI are composed of paramagnetic materials, or elements with unpaired electrons having, therefore, intrinsic magnetic dipole moments. Of these, the most widely used are based on gadolinium, an ion of the lanthanide series, chelated by means of ligation with, for instance, diethylene triamine pentaacetic acid (Gd-DTPA), in order to eliminate its highly toxic effect. Once injected into a peripheral vein at doses of 0.1–0.2 mmol/kg, Gd-DTPA acts as an intravascular agent, although rapidly distributed throughout the extracellular compartment of tissues, similarly to iodinated contrast agents, and exhibiting a plasma half-life of 20 minutes. Gd-DTPA is a T1 enhancing agent that shortens the T1 relaxation time of tissues where it is distributed, increasing their signal intensity with T1-sensitive imaging sequences.

Replacement of Gd with dysprosium in the same DTPA chelate induces the so-called magnetic susceptibility effect, which diminishes or eliminates the signal intensity from contrasted tissues, this causing a decrease in T2 relaxation time with signal loss on T2-sensitive imaging sequences. Susceptibility agents are not commercially available for clinical use at the present time.

Contrast agents are useful in 3 areas of cardiovascular MRI: (1) as intravascular agents in MR angiography (MRA); (2) to assess their uptake by a specific structure, such as abnormal cardiac or paracardiac masses; and (3) to detect its presence and distribution through the myocardium in the diagnostic assessment of ischemic heart disease.

A true sub-specialty of MRI in itself, MRA will not be treated here. The reader may obtain useful practical information from various excellent sources dedicated to the technique[1,2].

9.2 Contrast Agents in the Study of Abnormal Cardiac and Paracardiac Masses

Cardiac abnormal masses of diverse origin are a relatively frequent finding in an MRI examination, mainly corresponding to intracardiac thrombus, mural or intracavitary tumors, or paracardiac cysts or hematomas. Their distinction from normal myocardium, particularly in the case of intramural tumors, may be equivocal because of the similarity of signal intensity between tumor and normal myocardium on conventional images.

Enhancement in the signal intensity on spin echo T1 of a particular abnormal mass after administration of Gd-DTPA indicates its solid vascularized nature[3], as occurs with cardiac[4] (Figure 9.1) or mediastinal[5] (Figure 9.2) tumors. In the case of intramural cardiac tumors, differences in vascularity and in the proportion of interstitial space between tumor and normal myocardium usually causes a differential enhancement after contrast that helps to delineate the tumor margins. Moreover, areas of less intense enhancement within the tumor have been correlated, in the case of atrial myxoma[6], with hystological changes of cystic or necrotic origin in the specimen where the contrast medium cannot accumulate. On the other hand, non-tumoral masses such as thrombus, pericardial cysts or mediastinal hematoma do not exhibit signal enhancement on contrasted images[7].

9.3 Contrast Agents in the Assessment of Ischemic Heart Disease

The outstanding role of ischemic heart disease in public health demands an exhaustive testing of all resources with potential usefulness in its management. Thus, a great deal of effort has been recently devoted to study the applications of MRI in the field and, particularly, to explore the potentially promising benefits of using contrast media. Properties of contrast agents seem particularly well suited to accomplish the main goals in the management of the patient with coronary artery disease: to assess myocardial perfusion, to quantify the extension of myocardial infarction, differentiating between occlusive and reperfused infarcts and, also, establishing potential viability of tissue[8]. Experimental studies have rendered stimulating results in all these areas, although its actual clinical value is still under investigation.

a. Myocardial perfusion

The more direct method for identifying potentially ischemic myocardium is perfusion imaging. The absence of differential spontaneous signal intensities on MRI between normal and ischemic myocardium in the acute phase of ischemia requires the use of contrast agents to highlight differences in the enhancement of normal and underperfused myocardial regions. Unlike nuclear tracers, which are trapped in the myocardium, MRI contrast agents distribute in the extracellular space and are rapidly excreted from the body. Also, eventual differences in regional myocardial enhancement between normal and ischemic areas can be seen only transiently, as contrast rapidly redistributes into ischemic regions, differences in regional enhancement being then lost. Thus, a monitoring of the early distribution of the agent during the first 1–2 minutes after injection is required (first pass technique). This prevents study of the transit of a bolus of contrast agent with conventional MRI acquisition techniques, but requires ultrafast gradient echo (GRE) or echo planar imaging (EPI), where images can be obtained in fractions of a second (subsecond imaging techniques)[9]. Current fast GRE techniques still have some inconveniences, such as a limited temporal resolution that permits the monitoring of only 1 to 3 tomographic levels in one heart beat. EPI techniques, although not widely available to date, need only 30 to 50 msec to completely acquire one image allowing the entire ventricle to be imaged within one heart beat[10].

First-pass study of Gd-DTPA using fast MR techniques allows the detection of signal enhancement first in the right ventricular

FIGURE 9.1 A and B

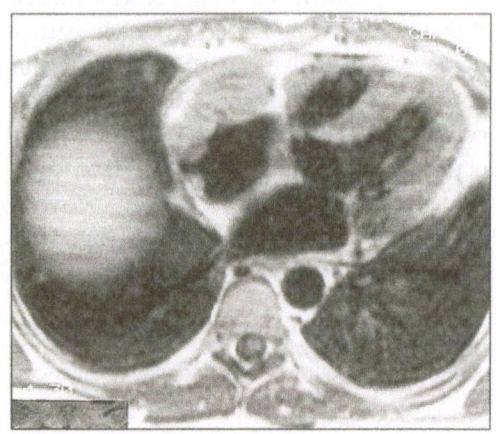 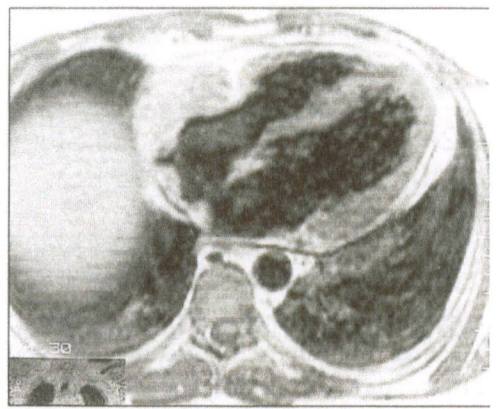

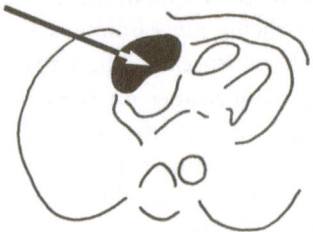 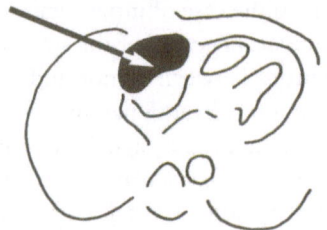

FIGURE 9.2 A and B

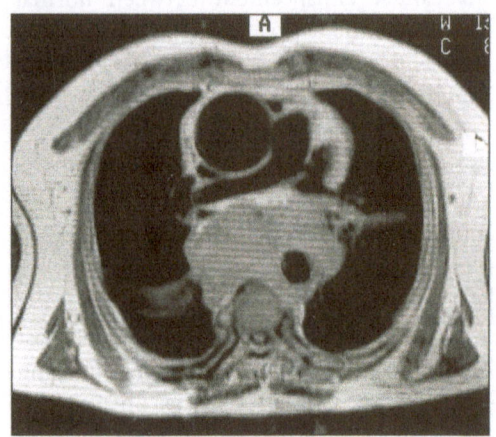 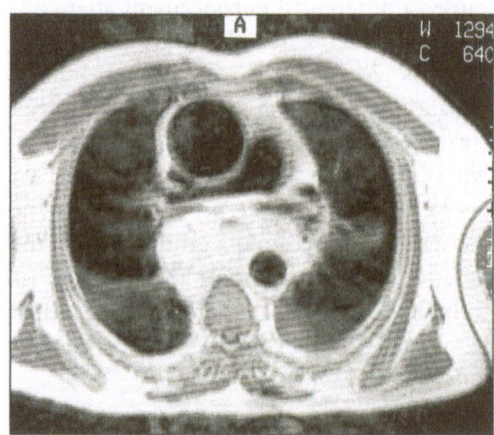

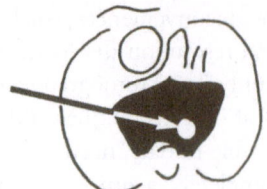 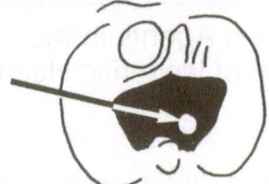

cavity and, then, in the left ventricle and finally at the myocardial level (Figure 9.3). By this method, lower peak signal intensity and lower rate of signal increase have been demonstrated in myocardial regions perfused by diseased vessels compared with that in myocardial segments dependent on normal coronary arteries in humans in the resting state[11]. The technique may also be performed after the administration of dypiridamole[12] to increase flow and volume causing a "steal phenomenon" in ischemic areas and thus inducing substantial heterogeneity of regional blood flow.

The measurement of myocardial perfusion is possible with this method by considering the peak myocardial enhancement if a linear relation between tracer concentration and signal enhancement is assumed. Although attempts to quantitate regional myocardial blood flow by deriving mean transit time from curves of signal intensity versus time have proved feasible[13], a generally accepted method of acquiring and analyzing MR perfusion images does not exist yet. Thus, the technique has not replaced nuclear methods, although some advantages of MRI are particularly promising, such as its higher resolution and potential for measurement of absolute values of myocardial blood perfusion.

b. Myocardial infarction

Unlike acute ischemia, the location and extent of acute and subacute infarction can be visualized on T2 weighted spin echo images as an area of increased signal intensity due to the formation of interstitial edema with an increase in myocardial relaxation times. T2 sequences, however, frequently induce flow artifacts in cardiac studies due to the long TR and TE required. Administration of contrast media enables the detection of recent infarction on T1 spin echo due to differences in wash-in and wash-out between normal and ischemic myocardium. The delayed arrival of contrast in the infarcted area and its

prolonged elimination allows detection of its presence when images are obtained between 20–30 minutes after the administration of contrast, once the agent has been washed from the normal myocardium (Figure 9.4). Only recent infarcts (<6 weeks) are able to be detected by this method[14], as the disappearance of interstitial edema and formation of fibrous scar in the area of chronic myocardial necrosis do not allow the contrast to be accumulated at this level. When the entire left ventricle is covered by a series of short axis slices (Figure 9.5), quantitation of the infarct size is possible by measuring enhanced areas on every slice (Figure 9.6) this allowing the calculation of the total infarcted mass of the left ventricle[15].

c. Patency of the infarct-related artery

An important point, in the era of thrombolysis and intervention in acute myocardial infarction, is the assessment of residual patency of the infarct related artery. Although, theoretically, in cases of acute infarction with an occluded artery, contrast should not diffuse into the necrotic region rendering a false-negative diagnosis, due to the possible presence of collateral flow with diffusion of the contrast agent into the center of the infarct and the long acquisition times allowing the display of the steady-state phase of contrast medium distribution, occluded and reperfused infarctions show apparently equal degrees of enhancement[16]. When measuring infarct sizes, however, it has been shown that these are significantly smaller in reperfused patients than in those with occluded arteries[17]. Later studies focused on the pattern of signal enhancement of the infarcted area have show that differences in homogeneity of enhancement may be seen[18] and that while virtually all patients with myocardial infarction exhibit an area of increased signal intensity within the infarcted region, uniform contrast hyperenhancement

F. 9.1. Transaxial spin echo images before (A) and after (B) gadolinium showing hyperenhancement of an intramural mass involving the right atrial wall (arrow). A diagnosis of hamangiosarcoma was made after surgical removal of the tumor.

F. 9.2. Transaxial spin echo images before (A) and after (B) gadolinium showing diffuse hyperenhancement of a large mass of the posterior mediastinum corresponding to a non-Hodgkin lymphoma, as proven by thoracoscopy-guided biopsy.

138

FIGURE 9.3

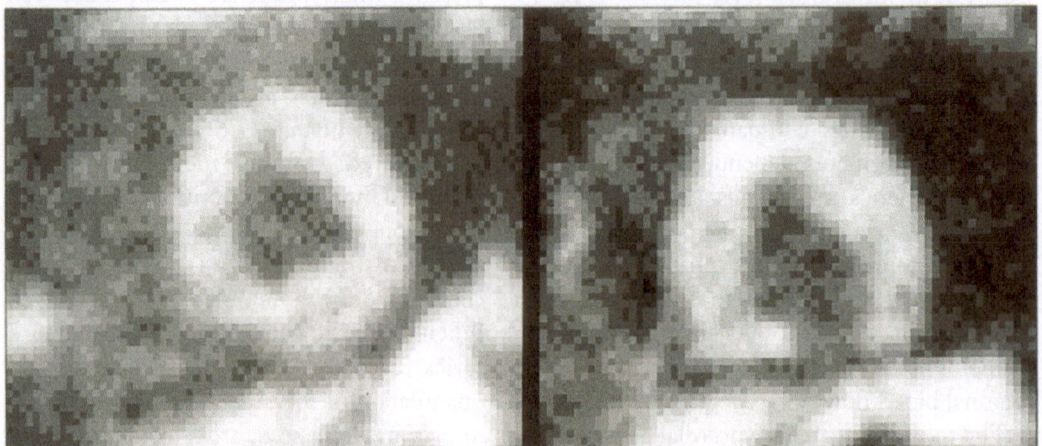

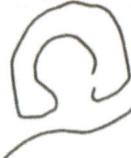 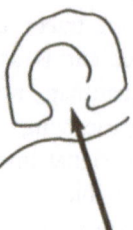

FIGURE 9.4 A and B

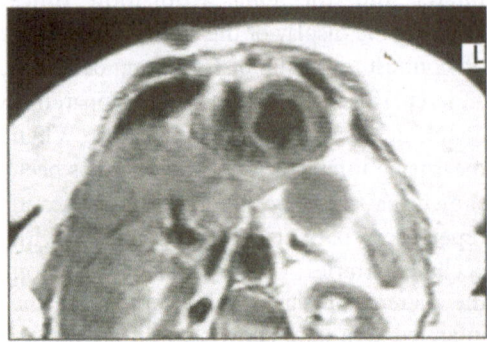 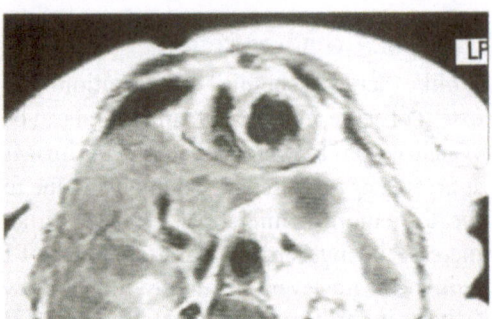

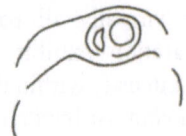 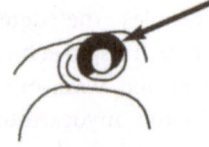

(Figures 9.4–9.6) is associated with patent infarct-related arteries, while the presence of a central hypoenhanced area ("doughnut pattern") (Figure 9.7) is seen in cases with coronary occlusion at angiography[19]. The study of "first pass" of a contrast agent by means of fast MRI sequences is also helpful in the assessment of vessel patency after acute infarction as cases with occlusion exhibit a slower wash-in of contrast in the infarct region leading to longer time-to-peak intensity and also a more delayed wash-out compared with patients with a patent artery[20]

d. Myocardial viability

The important issue of establishing the presence of potentially reversible myocardial damage after infarction has also been addressed in studies using contrast MRI agents. Evidence that the administration of Gd-DTPA enhances reperfused reversibly injured myocardium to a degree equivalent to that of normal myocardium has prompted the investigation of susceptibility enhancing agents such as dysprosium, which has the property of diffusing throughout the intracellular compartment in reperfused myocardial regions and, thus, may be helpful in identifying viable myocardium[8]. The method, however, has not been validated in human studies. More recent clinical reports[21] have shown that, again, the pattern of enhancement of the infarcted zone by gadolinium on conventional spin echo sequences is useful in practice to assess tissue viability. Thus, subendocardial or absent infarct enhancement patterns have a high positive predictive value for viability while homogeneous transmural enhancement (Figures 9.4–9.6) correlates with the absence of functional recovery only in nearly half of infarct segments and, finally, the pattern of signal enhancement surrounding a region without signal ("doughnut") (Figure 9.7) is exclusively associated with the absence of

viability. Similarly, other studies[18] have shown that a pattern of transmural and marginal enhancement (Figure 9.8) also suggests extensive myocardial infarction with infarct expansion and less viable myocardium. If confirmed in larger studies, these findings would have interesting clinical implications in the selection of patients in whom a further investigation (i.e. contractile reserve determination with dobutamine echocardiography or MRI) is worth performing in order to demonstrate myocardial viability.

Thus, a relevant role of MRI in conjunction with contrast agents may be envisaged in the near future for the management of ischemic heart disease, particularly when the method is seen as an adjunct to the other capabilities of MRI, such as for studying ventricular structure and function, this providing the cardiologist with an attractively complete tool for a comprehensive study in these patients[22]. Despite these promising expectations, however, further solid clinical evidence will be necessary for MRI to be considered as a first line imaging method in ischemic diseases[23], probably, in part, due to the proven usefulness in practice of other current diagnostic techniques.

References

1. Raymond HW, Zwiebel WJ, Swartz JD, eds. Vascular imaging with CT and MR. Semin Ultrasound CT MR 1996; 17: 279–411.

2. Prince MR, Grist TM, Debatin JF, eds. 3D Contrast MR Angiography. New York, Springer; 1997.

3. Brasch RC, Weinmann HJ, Wesbey GE. Contrast-enhanced NMR imaging: animal studies using gadolinium-DTPA complex. Am J Roentgenol AJR 1984; 142: 625–30.

4. Funari M, Fujita N, Peck WW, Higgins CB. Cardiac tumors: assessment with Gd-DTPA

F. 9.3. Left ventricular short axis views of a T1-weighted spin echo EPI study obtained during the first pass of a gadolinium-DTPA bolus injection at peak wash-in at rest (left panel) and during stress (right panel). A perfusion defect of the inferior wall is seen in the stress study (arrow). (Courtesy of JR Panting, PD Gatehouse, GZ Yang, DN Firmin, and DJ Pennell, from the Royal Brompton Hospital, London).

F. 9.4. Basal (A) and contrast-enhanced (B) spin echo ventricular short-axis images at the basal level in a case of large transmural anterior myocardial infarction (arrow).

FIGURE 9.5 A & B

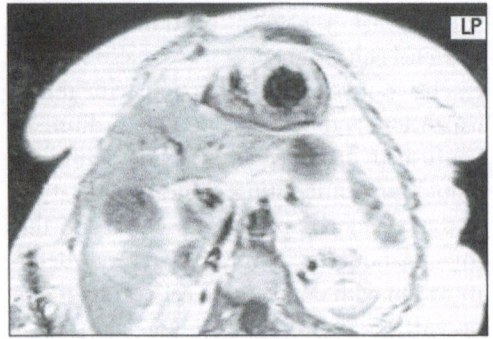

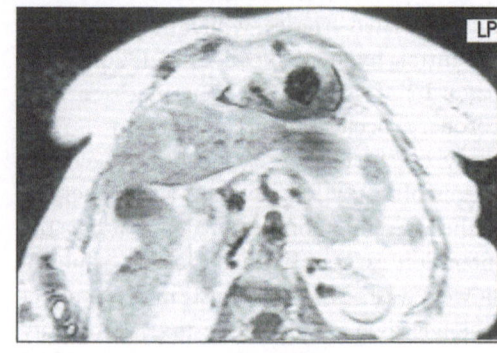

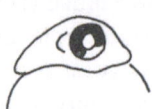

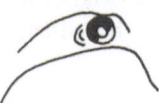

FIGURE 9.6

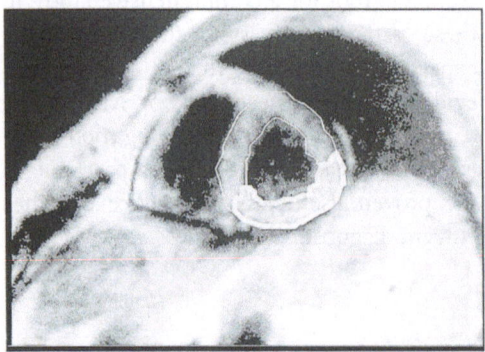

FIGURE 9.8

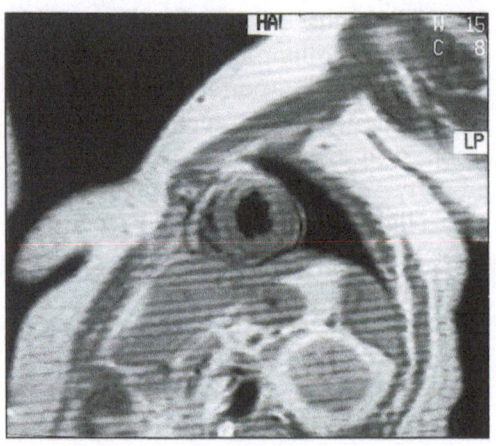

FIGURE 9.7

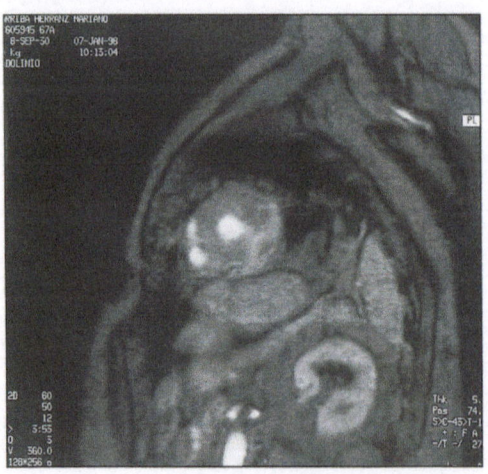

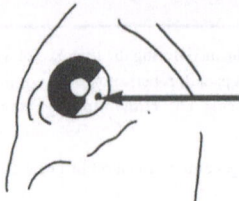

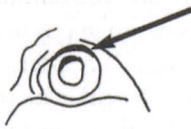

F. 9.5. Contrasted short-axis slices from the same case presented in Figure 9.4, showing transmural enhancement of the anterior left ventricular wall also at the medial (A) end apical (B) levels.

F. 9.6. Manual planimetry of the contrast enhanced area of a posterior left ventricular infarction allowing the measurement of its extension in relation to the whole cross sectional myocardial area in this particular slice.

F. 9.7. Short-axis gradient echo image showing a gadolinium study in a case of recent infarction of the left ventricular posterior wall; a "doughnut" pattern of enhancement is seen, where an area of increased signal intensity surrounds a central zone (arrow) of hypo-enhancement.

F. 9.8. Short-axis spin echo image in a patient with anterior infarction showing a pattern of transmural contrast enhancement with particularly high signal intensity at both the endocardial and epicardial margins (arrow).

enhanced MR imaging. J Comput Assist Tomogr 1991; 15: 953–8.

5. Forsgren G, Nyman R, Glimelius B, Hagberg H, Rehn S, Hemmingsson A. Gd-DTPA-enhanced MR imaging in mediastinal Hodgkin's disease. Acta Radiol 1994; 35: 564–9.

6. Matsuoka H, Hamada M, Honda T, et al. Morphologic and histologic characterization of cardiac myxomas by magnetic resonance imaging. Angiology 1996; 47: 693–8

7. Semelka RC, Shoenut JP, Wilson ME, Pellech AE, Patton JN. Cardiac masses: signal intensity features on spin-echo, gradient-echo, gadolinium-enhanced spin-echo, and TurboFLASH images. J Magn Reson Imaging 1992; 2: 415–20.

8. Saeed M, Wendland MF, Higgins CB. Contrast media for MR imaging of the heart. J Magn Reson Imaging 1994; 4: 269–79.

9. Pettigrew R, Oshinski J, Dixon WT. Magnetic resonance imaging techniques for assessing myocardial perfusion. In: Higgins CB, Ingwall JS, Pohost GM, eds. Current and future applications of magnetic resonance in cardiovascular disease. New York: Futura; 1998: 37–52.

10. Crnac J, Schmidt MC, Theissen P, Sechtem U. Assessment of myocardial perfusion by magnetic resonance imaging. Herz 1997; 22: 16–28.

11. Manning WJ, Atkinson DJ, Grossman W, Paulin S, Edelman RR. First-pass nuclear magnetic resonance imaging studies using gadolinium-DTPA in patients with coronary artery disease. J Am Coll Cardiol 1991; 18: 959–65.

12. Schaefer S, van Tyen R, Saloner D. Evaluation of myocardial perfusion abnormalities with gadolinium-enhanced snapshot MR imaging in humans. Work in progress. Radiology 1992; 185: 795–801.

13. Keijer JT, van Rossum AC, van Eenige MJ, et al. Semiquantitation of regional myocardial blood flow in normal human subjects by first-pass magnetic resonance imaging. Am Heart J 1995; 130: 893–901.

14. van Dijkman PR, van der Wall EE, de Roos A, et al. Acute, subacute, and chronic myocardial infarction: quantitative analysis of gadolinium-enhanced MR images. Radiology 1991; 180: 147–51.

15. Holman ER, van Jonbergen HP, van Dijkman PR, van der Laarse A, de Roos A, van der Wall EE. Comparison of magnetic resonance imaging studies with enzymatic indexes of myocardial necrosis for quantification of myocardial infarct size. Am J Cardiol 1993; 71: 1036–40.

16. Van Rossum AC, Visser FC, Van Eenige MJ, et al. Value of gadolinium-diethylene-triamine penta-acetic acid dynamics in magnetic resonance imaging of acute myocardial infarction with occluded and reperfused coronary arteries after thrombolysis. Am J Cardiol 1990; 65: 845–51.

17. de Roos A, Matheijssen NA, Doornbos J, van Dijkman PR, van Voorthuisen AE, van der Wall EE. Myocardial infarct size after reperfusion therapy: assessment with Gd-DTPA-enhanced MR imaging. Radiology 1990; 176: 517–21.

18. Yokota C, Nonogi H, Miyazaki S, et al. Gadolinium-enhanced magnetic resonance imaging in acute myocardial infarction. Am J Cardiol 1995; 75: 577–81.

19. Lima JA, Judd RM, Bazille A, Schulman SP, Atalar E, Zerhouni EA. Regional heterogeneity of human myocardial infarcts demonstrated by contrast-enhanced MRI. Potential mechanisms. Circulation 1995; 92: 1117–25.

20. Dendale P, Franken PR, Meusel M, van der Geest R, de Roos A. Distinction between open and occluded infarct-related arteries using contrast-enhanced magnetic resonance imaging. Am J Cardiol 1997; 80: 334–6.

21. Dendale P, Franken PR, Block P, Pratikakis Y, De Roos A. Contrast enhanced and functional magnetic resonance imaging for the detection of viable myocardium after infarction. Am Heart J 1998; 135: 875–80.

22. Kramer CM, Rogers WJ, Geskin G, et al. Usefulness of magnetic resonance imaging early after acute myocardial infarction. Am J Cardiol 1997; 80: 690–5.

23. The clinical role of magnetic resonance in cardiovascular disease. Task Force of the European Society of Cardiology, in collaboration with the Association of European Paediatric Cardiologists. Eur Heart J 1998; 19: 19–39.

Library of Congress Cataloging-in-Publication data is available.

ISBN 978-94-010-5931-2   ISBN 978-94-011-4544-2 (eBook)
DOI 10.1007/978-94-011-4544-2

Printed on acid-free paper